FAMILY PERSPECTIVES ON BED WETTING IN YOUNG PEOPLE

For my parents, Morris and Joy

Family perspectives on bed wetting in young people

MOYA J MORISON
Formerly Department of Health and Nursing
Queen Margaret College
Edinburgh

Avebury

Aldershot • Brookfield USA • Hong Kong • Singapore • Sydney

Published by
Avebury
Ashgate Publishing Limited
Gower House
Croft Road
Aldershot
Hants GU11 3HR
England

Ashgate Publishing Company
Old Post Road
Brookfield
Vermont 05036
USA

British Library Cataloguing in Publication Data

Morison, Moya J.
    Family perspectives on bed wetting in young people
    1. Enuresis 2. Enuresis - Social aspects 3. Pediatric urology
    4. Family
    I. Title
    618 . 9 ' 2849

    ISBN 1 85972 346 2

Library of Congress Catalog Card Number: 96-83219

Printed and bound by Athenaeum Press, Ltd.,
Gateshead, Tyne & Wear.

Contents

Figures and tables

Foreword

A nurse's perspective

It is a privilege to be associated with this valuable addition to nursing knowledge.

Bed wetting in young people has, to date, not generated the same measure of academic interest or human concern as life-threatening, degenerative or acute disease conditions. However, as the author, who conducted the research shows, it constitutes a problem that can seriously diminish the quality of life of the young person as well as that of his or her family. The research identified "perceived helplessness" as a key issue, permeating the whole system and often activating a downward spiral leading to the abdication of effort and responsibility by the young people themselves, by their parents and sometimes by health care professionals. In this way, alone, the work makes a significant contribution to our understanding of the problem.

More than that, the research reported in this book stands out in several ways, of which only two can be mentioned here. The first is the creativity in thinking which influenced the researcher's approach and the second, the scientific rigour which gave the creativity "academic credence". It is a superb example of a human problem, identified, opened up and seriously studied.

Although the researcher came to the problem from a quantitative research tradition, she recognised the need to allow her subjects, children and adults, to explain in their own words and in other ways what the problem of bed wetting meant to them. She saw the need for a mainly ethnographic qualitative perspective. Moreover, a way had to be found by which the feelings of children, whose linguistic skills were not adequate, could be captured. The researcher soon became aware that the problem of bed wetting in young people, aged 5 to 20 years, was a family problem, rather than an individual one, thereby contributing significantly to the rapidly increasing domain of family nursing. Although the research was descriptive in design and, therefore, has no prescriptive power, its message to health visitors and other health professionals is loud and clear. Having been a practising health visitor myself, I would have derived great benefit from research findings just to alert me to such a huge and largely hidden problem. As a researcher I welcome the ingenious blend of different approaches and data collection methods, such as the use of faces to indicate feelings which could not be expressed verbally.

Nursing, which includes health visiting, is a complex and unique professional activity. As such, it requires complex and unique methods to explore it. This study shows how such an abstract normative statement can be translated into a living reality with its limitless potential for generating badly needed new knowledge.

Lisbeth Hockey   OBE, PhD, FRCN, Hon FRCGP
Visiting Professor, Buckinghamshire College of Brunel University
Honorary Reader in Nursing, Queen Margaret College, Edinburgh

A urologist's perspective

It is refreshing to encounter a writer who can combine the qualities of a caring and dedicated observer with the analytical skill demonstrated in the detailed review and application of the scientific research tools. The caring element is expressed in plain language, making use of quotations from young bed wetters and members of their families. At first glance, the language of the scientific sections is less attractive to the average medical or nurse clinician unaccustomed to scientific "jargon". Persevere. This is not jargon, rather it is the language necessary for the explanation of the analytical approach leading to constructive proposals for future research, and of more immediate importance, a well reasoned outline of attainable improvements to current practice. Moya Morison has described concepts that are new to me.

As a urologist with over 25 years deep interest in the prevention, investigation and management of urinary incontinence, I agree that young people who wet the bed are best assessed in the family setting, and that is best done by the primary health care team. The need for a multidisciplinary approach is emphasised, as is the need for each member of the team to recognise the limits of their expertise and be prepared to involve others. The author refers to the fragmented and poorly supported provision of professional help, and to the lack of awareness that the management of bed wetting "can be a prolonged and difficult professional engagement". Examples are given of the professional exhausting their limited therapeutic repertoire, their sense of failure deepening that of the young bed wetter and family.

Clearly professionals need better training and support. There are several national and international organisations active in the field of incontinence, such as the International Continence Society, Association for Continence Advice, the Continence Foundation, and the Enuresis Resource and Information Centre. I am sure all will agree that we need more health care professionals of this researcher's calibre to address the issue, and to assist in training the trainers, if not the professionals in the field.

This monograph merits a wide audience, the scientific concepts reaching far beyond the topic of bed wetting.

Eric Glen FRCS
Consultant Urological Surgeon, Southern General Hospital, Glasgow
Founder and past President of the International Continence Society

A general practitioner's perspective

I am delighted to have been asked to write one of the Forewords to this research monograph on bed wetting in young people.

Enuresis is a complex problem involving subtle interactions not only within the family, but between the family and health professionals. Two of the problems for health professionals have been that bed wetting is often hidden and therefore underestimated, and secondly because it has been difficult to define the age at which a diagnosis is appropriate. Dismissal of parental concern with the words "he or she will grow out of it" gives just as wrong a message as immediate intervention with either drugs such as antidepressants or antidiuretic hormone, or the application of behavioural methods such as pad and alarm.

Until recently the scientific training of doctors and nurses has eschewed qualitative research and relied on quantitative approaches and controlled randomised trials. The current fashion in medicine is for evidence based guidelines and protocols. However, failure to undertake good qualitative research can mean a failure to develop appropriate hypotheses. Moya Morison's detailed and careful evaluation of 20 young people in 19 families leads us into a world of "learned helplessness" which pervades the entire family. It would be my hope that in reading this monograph other professionals will be stimulated into addressing the research and management issues which it raises.

Richard Simpson FRCPsych
Forth Valley Primary Care Research Group
Honorary Professor, Department of Psychology, Stirling University

Acknowledgements

This study, and this account of it, have been made possible by the goodwill, help and encouragement of so many people. Special thanks are due to the families who shared their experiences and feelings with me over several occasions and to my husband Graeme and my parents-in-law Helen and Alastair who have lived with this study for three years and helped in innumerable ways. They cheerfully and tirelessly typed the PhD thesis, upon which this monograph is based and learned many new computing skills to facilitate its presentation. It was a privilege and an honour to have Lisbeth Hockey as a supervisor of the study. She is the best teacher that I have ever known. I have received helpful comments and support from so many staff within Forth Valley Health Board, especially from Richard Simpson and Irene Linton. I am particularly grateful to the health visitors who helped with the enrolment of the families and shared their experiences of helping families with a bed wetting child, and to the members of the GP Research Group (now Primary Care Research Group) who offered constructive comments on the study's design and on the contents of the supplementary data collection tools. The help of George McKelvie with the design and analysis of the urinary symptoms questionnaire and his comments on the study's findings, from a urologist's perspective, has proved invaluable. My sincere thanks also go to Dorothy Whyte for introducing me to the family systems nursing literature and for inspiring me, through her example, to write this monograph. I would also like to thank Helen Morison and Valerie Chuter who willingly undertook the onerous task of conversation transcription, Francine Cheater and Phil Runciman for their helpful comments and the Coloplast Charitable Trust for a grant towards the cost of the audio-recording equipment. To all those who have helped me, whether or not specifically mentioned here, I would like to extend my warmest thanks.

Introduction

No other complaint [bed wetting] has given rise to so many treatment endeavours and such dispute as to its pathogenesis and whether it can properly be characterised as a disease or not. Treatment ranges from ritual procedures to modern medical treatment with a solid scientific basis. Some specialists consider the complaint to be a variation of normality, whereas others regard it as a disease. Regardless of whether one subscribes to one opinion or the other, modern urbanised life puts demands on children at an early age to be able to control continence in order to comply socially.

Djurhuus, Norgaard and Rittig (1992) p.8

Bed wetting is a phenomenon surrounded by both mystery and controversy. It has been described as a benign, self-limiting pathology whose natural course (to dryness) can be accelerated by treatment and as a social construct, that is as deviance from socially accepted norms regarding the age at which a child should be reliably dry at night. In the latter approach a bed wetting child is defined not so much as having a pathophysiological problem but as failing to meet society's expectations of the age of attainment of a normal developmental milestone.

In recent times, the cause of bed wetting has been variously attributed to reduced bladder capacity, unstable bladder contractions, bladder outlet disturbances, sleep disorders, urine output regulation dysfunction or psychological problems. The focus of much clinical research has been on bladder function and there have been many clinical trials of interventions which are based on the belief that bed wetting is a pathophysiological problem.

The interventions have included pharmacologically reducing the rate and volume of urine production overnight, pharmacotherapy aimed at reducing

1

unstable bladder contractions and various surgical interventions to correct supposed bladder outlet disturbances. Successful treatment with the antidiuretic hormone arginine vasopressin (AVP) suggests that night time polyuria and AVP deficiency may contribute to bed wetting but many other therapeutic approaches still in use are said to be of questionable efficacy (Norgaard, 1991; Wille, 1994).

There is a growing body of evidence that bed wetting involves a normal, complete micturition which can occur at any stage in the sleep cycle, in young people who are psychologically normal and who have a normal bladder capacity (where the bed wetting is monosymptomatic). There is, however, some evidence that the bed wetting child's arousal response to a full bladder may be underdeveloped or malfunctioning.

Over the last 50 years one of the most successful treatment approaches for monosymptomatic bed wetters has been behavioural training using a bedside or body worn alarm (Forsythe and Butler, 1989). The rationale behind this method is that the young person needs to learn to wake up to the physiological signals that the bladder is full.

An organic cause for bed wetting, such as a congenital abnormality or a neurological disorder, is only identified in a very small percentage of cases. The aetiology of bed wetting for the majority of monosymptomatic bed wetters is almost certainly multifactorial and it is still a matter of considerable debate.

At the heart of the controversy is the very practical question: "Whose business is it?" Many professionals regard the treatment of bed wetting as being within their remit, including urologists, paediatricians, clinical psychologists, general practitioners (GPs) and nurses. In the first instance parents may seek help from their GP or their health visitor. In other cases the health visitor may discover the young person's bed wetting at a pre-school check or when visiting the family at home for another purpose, or it may be discovered by the school nurse. After ruling out obvious congenital abnormalities, neurological disorders or other possible causes such as repeated urinary tract infections, the GP may refer the young person to a paediatrician, a urologist or a clinical psychologist for a specialist opinion. Urologists describe bed wetting as the most common "urological" complaint in children (Djurhuus et al, 1992), yet there is no consensus among them or among paediatricians about how best to treat it. The diversity of treatment approaches in current use seems to add to the uncertainty about what it is that is actually being treated.

While many health care professionals may become involved with some families at one time or another in their search for a solution to the young person's bed wetting, there is evidence to suggest that many families rarely if ever actively seek help from any health care professional (Devlin, 1991; Foxman et al, 1986). It has been estimated that 500,000 young people in the UK wet the bed on some occasions (Blackwell, 1995) yet the problem is, for the most part, hidden and many sufferers believe themselves to be alone.

There is a growing body of anecdotal evidence, collected by community based nurses and clinical psychologists running specialist enuresis clinics, that both the young person and the family feel embarrassment at the young person's failure to attain a developmental milestone which the majority of children attain between the ages of three and four years. These anecdotal accounts suggest that bed wetting can have far reaching consequences for the young person and the family.

As bed wetting is for the most part managed by the family, within the context of every day family life, it seemed that an understanding of how families experience and respond to a young person's bed wetting, and their experience of methods suggested by health care professionals, could have implications for both service organisation and service delivery.

An over view of the study

The aim of the study, as initially envisaged, was to explore the nature and experience of bed wetting from the perspective of young people who wet the bed, and that of their parents and siblings. A qualitative, inductive approach was used which allowed the study's participants to explain in their own words and in other ways what the problem of bed wetting meant to them. Underlying the approach taken was the assumption that there could be concepts pertaining to the phenomenon of bed wetting that had yet to be discovered, or at least articulated in a coherent way.

Nineteen families and twenty young people aged 4 to 17 years, living in some of the most deprived as well as the most affluent localities in the study area, took part. The principal method of data gathering was in depth interviewing, conducted over a period of two to three months for each family.

In depth interviewing of children and adolescents can be challenging. In recognition of the limits imposed by the children's cognitive, social and linguistic skills and in anticipation that some young people might be too ashamed about their lack of night time bladder control to be able to speak freely about it with a stranger, the young people were encouraged to express their feelings through drawings and with the aid of "faces-feelings" cards. These methods proved helpful in facilitating communication and the results were illuminating.

In addition to the in depth interviews with families, three supplementary

3

methods of data collection were incorporated into the study's design for specific purposes. These were: a urinary symptoms questionnaire, completed by the family before the researcher's first visit; diaries, in which the young person and his or her principal carer recorded events over a one month period as they actually happened, and a checklist of the methods used by families to encourage the young person's bed wetting to stop, completed by the researcher in consultation with the family at the conclusion of the last visit.

By combining both qualitative and quantitative approaches and methods in a fully integrated way, a clearer understanding of the meaning of bed wetting has been gained, from the family's perspective, than could have been achieved using one approach alone.

Analysis of the interview transcripts was facilitated by NUD•IST Power Version 3.0 computer software. With the aid of memos, logic diagrams and a coding paradigm (axial coding) the relationships between emergent concepts were identified and tested and a grounded theory developed around the core concept of "perceived control", which usually manifested as "perceived helplessness".

The study has revealed many insights into family processes and the roles played by individual family members, including fathers and siblings. Several conditions have been identified which may need to be fulfilled for the young person to have the best chance of becoming reliably dry at night, using conventional treatment methods. It is argued that the family, rather than the individual or the mother-child dyad, should be the unit of any therapeutic intervention.

An overview of the monograph

The material in this monograph is arranged in six chapters. Chapter 1 summarises the findings of the literature review undertaken before and during the early stages of data collection. Chapter 2 outlines and justifies the study's design and methods. Chapter 3 sets the scene for the remaining chapters by summarising contextual data about the families enrolled into the study. Chapter 4 seeks to answer the initial broad research questions by describing the families' experiences of living with a young person who wets the bed. Chapter 5 describes family members' beliefs about and attitudes towards bed wetting and explores the relationship between beliefs, feelings and behaviour as family members interact with one another from day to day. This chapter includes an analysis of the concepts of perceived helplessness and perceived control. Chapter 6 outlines the implications of this study's findings for practice and indicates some directions for further research.

1 The literature review

Many times ... as well old men as children, are oftentimes annoied, wha their urine issueth out either in their slepe or waking against their willes, havi(n)g no power to reteine it whan it cometh ...

Phaire (1553/1957) p.53

This chapter begins by summarising the findings of a literature review on bed wetting. It includes a discussion of the nature of bed wetting and its prevalence, the management of bed wetting by families and by health care professionals and the impact of bed wetting on the individual and the family. This is followed by a brief review of the literature on the nature of the family and the dynamics of the interaction of family members. The chapter ends by highlighting some unanswered questions about bed wetting and its management, which are of particular relevance to this study.

What is bed wetting?

Bed wetting is a phenomenon whose cause is uncertain. Even in recent times it has been attributed to reduced bladder capacity, unstable bladder contractions, bladder outlet disturbances, sleep disorders, urine output regulation dysfunction or psychological problems (Norgaard, 1991). An organic cause for bed wetting, such as a congenital abnormality or a neurogenic disorder, is only identified in a very small percentage of cases. The aetiology of bed wetting for the majority of monosymptomatic bed wetters is still a matter of considerable controversy within the medical profession, and between health care professionals and social scientists more generally and it is almost certainly multifactorial.

5

A review of the literature on bed wetting, undertaken before contact was made with families, uncovered two contrasting perspectives. In the medical literature bed wetting is often described as a benign self-limiting pathology, whose natural course (to dryness) can be accelerated by treatment. However, it is generally not, now regarded as a distinct disease or disorder but as a symptom (Vereecken, 1990).

A contrasting perspective is to describe bed wetting as a social construct, that is as deviance from socially accepted norms regarding the age at which a young person should be reliably dry at night (Leenders, 1993). In the latter approach, a bed wetting child is defined not so much as having a pathophysiological problem but as failing to meet society's expectations of the age of attainment of a normal developmental milestone.

In practice many health care professionals straddle these contrasting perspectives by defining bed wetting in socio-medical terms.

The perspective brought to bed wetting by any professional working with a family influences how bed wetting is defined and the overall approach adopted to the problem, as well as influencing any specific treatment prescribed. Whether a professional acknowledges and is prepared to address the social and emotional consequences of bed wetting for the child and his or her family, or merely regards bed wetting as a benign self-limiting condition, can affect both the professional's attitude to the family and how seriously and quickly a solution to the problem is sought.

A study by Shelov et al (1981) suggests that parents expect their child to be dry at night at about the time that most children normally achieve dryness (between the ages of three and four years). Many parents become concerned about the bed wetting from then on, while most doctors do not define bed wetting as a problem until the child is considerably older than this. Clinicians may defer treatment until the child is seven years of age (or even older), believing that by this time the situation will, in most cases, have resolved itself.

Children are born unable to control bladder emptying voluntarily. They have to learn to void urine in a socially appropriate place and at a socially appropriate time, both in the day and at night (Norton, 1986). The acquisition of continence is said to be a complex skill which occurs early in childhood and which probably involves both spontaneous physiological maturation and the learning of certain associated social skills (Smith & Smith, 1987a, b). The dilemma, even for those health care professionals who adopt a socio-medical perspective, is to decide on the point at which wetting the bed becomes abnormal. The ways in which some health care professionals and researchers have defined urinary incontinence in childhood, and bed wetting in particular, are discussed in this context.

In a treatment manual written for professionals, a psychologist and a psychiatrist defined nocturnal enuresis as:

> ... persistent childhood bed wetting, which occurs in the absence of any discernible neurological or urological pathology, and which continues beyond an age by which most children, without the need for special attention, have gained normal control over functioning of the bladder.
>
> Bollard and Nettelbeck (1989) p.1

In a book written for parents, professionals and the older bed-wetting child the Deputy Director of Social Services in Oxfordshire, who has been involved in research into enuresis since the early 1970s, defined bed wetting very similarly as:

> ... persistent and frequent urination during sleep at an age at which a greater degree of night-time bladder control is considered to be normal.
>
> Morgan (1988) p.27

These definitions beg three important questions: from what age should wetting the bed be considered to be abnormal; how frequently does bed wetting need to occur to be defined as abnormal, and who decides?

There is considerable disagreement in the literature and amongst health care professionals about the answers to these questions.

Some researchers suggest that the physiological maturation needed for night time bladder control is present in children by the age of three, define bed wetting as a problem in individuals aged three and over and treat children for it from this age (Azrin et al, 1974). Others define nocturnal enuresis as: "over age four" (Devlin, 1991) or "at or after the age of five" (e.g. Forsythe and Butler, 1989; Hjälmås, 1992).

Forsythe and Butler's (1989, p.879) definition of enuresis is:

> ... involuntary discharge of urine by day or night or both, in a child aged five years or older, in the absence of congenital or acquired defects of the nervous system or urinary tract.

This is the definition used in publications originating from the Enuresis Resource and Information Centre (ERIC) at Bristol, such as their guide to enuresis, written for professionals (Blackwell, 1989, 1995) and their guidelines on minimum standards of practice in the treatment of enuresis

(Morgan, 1993), which were supported by the National Enuresis Research Steering Group. Their choice of the age of five years or older as defining enuresis corresponds to Hjälmås' (1992) more general proposal to define childhood urinary incontinence as occurring from five years of age. This is why "age five or over" was originally used as one of the inclusion criteria for this study.

Turning to the second question "how frequent does bed wetting need to be to be defined as abnormal?", frequencies quoted in the literature vary from seven nights a week to one night in six months (Jarvelin et al, 1990). Between these extremes definitions have included: "at least twice a week" (Devlin and O'Cathain, 1990); "at least once a week" (Couchells et al, 1981; Hjälmås, 1992); "at least once a month" (Devlin, 1991; Jarvelin et al, 1991; Oppel et al, 1968a) and "at least once in three months" (Foxman et al, 1986; Hellstrom et al, 1990).

In an extensive review of the pathophysiology of bed wetting Norgaard (1991, p.11) states:

> A clear-cut definition of nocturnal enuresis has never been given [in the literature], however when comparing the observed prevalence in the different studies we see almost the same in each age group. This indicates that a child who voids during sleep is an enuretic and that the severity of the problem varies from once a month to every night. The question as to when enuresis is to be considered pathological must be a matter of when the child or parents cross an iatrothropic limit.

Norgaard is suggesting that bed wetting becomes a problem when the parents and the child say it is, rather than at some arbitrary age and with some arbitrary frequency decided on by health care professionals. Norgaard's perspective is the one which came to be adopted in this study.

This is not to say that it is inappropriate for researchers to decide on operational definitions of bed wetting which involve a specification of the age of the children to be included and the minimum frequency of bed wetting (wet nights per week or month). However, such criteria should be decided in relation to the purpose of the study. Butler (1991), for example, has suggested a set of standard definitions to be used in research into the outcomes of trials of treatment efficacy.

Primary and secondary bed wetting

A distinction is often made in the literature between primary and secondary bed wetting but there is no universal agreement on the criteria to be used to

8

differentiate between them. According to Forsythe and Redmond (1974, p.259):

Primary nocturnal enuresis refers to the child who has never been dry at night and secondary or acquired nocturnal enuresis refers to the child who has been dry for at least a year before the onset of enuresis.

They do not specify a lower age limit. In another study Fergusson et al (1990, p.54) used the criteria of the American Psychiatric Association's Diagnostic and Statistical Manual of Mental Disorders (DSM3) which defines secondary bed wetting as:

The onset of bedwetting after the age of 5 years following at least 1 year during which the child had remained dry at night.

Other researchers have reduced to six months the length of time for which the child has to have been dry before being classified as having a secondary problem (eg. Devlin, 1991; Hjälmås, 1992; Jarvelin et al, 1990, 1991).

Cross-cultural perspectives

To shed some light on the cultural aspects of bed wetting, it is perhaps helpful to comment briefly upon the few cross-cultural studies that have been reported, such as Abramovitch and Abramovitch, 1989; Bose, 1992; Butler and Golding, 1986; de Jonge, 1973; Karandikar, 1992. In these studies bed wetting has been defined in many different ways. The prevalence rates quoted vary considerably, but they all suggest that the age at which a child is expected to be dry at night is culturally determined and can vary considerably in different cultures. Evidence from a health visitor involved with this study suggests that in another culture in the Far East, where the climate is warmer and the practical consequences of bed wetting are much easier to manage, wetting the bed is not a cause of anxiety and tension between mother and child and the age of attainment of day and night time bladder control is not an issue. In this Far Eastern culture the achievement of many other developmental milestones, such as the child's first tooth, first words and first attempts at walking, are noted and talked about with as much interest as they are by parents in the UK.

Towards a more pragmatic view of bed wetting

It is argued throughout this monograph that both the social and the medical

9

perspectives on bed wetting have merits in terms of what each highlights. However each approach also has deficiencies in terms of what is under-played or ignored. An understanding of both perspectives is important for clinical practice, especially for members of the primary health care team who may have a responsibility for the assessment and support of the child and his or her family over quite prolonged periods in childhood, perhaps extending into adolescence or even adulthood, in a minority of cases.

The epidemiology of bed wetting

Bed wetting is often thought of as a condition of childhood, yet it can affect some people into adolescence and even into their adult life. This section reviews what is known about the prevalence of bed wetting, the frequency of its occurrence for individuals (expressed as affected nights per week or month) and the proportion of bed wetters who also have day time urinary problems.

What proportion of the population wet the bed?

The lack of a universally accepted definition of bed wetting and the lack of agreement on the criteria for differentiating between primary and secondary bed wetting makes a meaningful comparison of the numerous epidemiological studies very difficult (e.g. Blomfield and Douglas, 1956; Devlin, 1991; Dodge et al, 1970; Foxman et al, 1986; Hellstrom et al, 1990; Jarvelin et al, 1988; Oppel et al, 1968a; Rutter et al, 1973; Verhulst et al, 1985). In a survey of the literature as long ago as 1973, de Jonge found that prevalence rates quoted for children varied from 1-40 per cent depending on the characteristics of the populations studied and how the researchers defined bed wetting.

However bed wetting is defined, it is generally accepted that it is a common problem which could be affecting as many as half a million children in the UK (Blackwell, 1995). Based on an average of two wet nights per week, it has been estimated that 15-20 per cent of 5 year olds, 7 per cent of 7 year olds, 5 per cent of 10 year olds, 2-3 per cent of 12 to 14 year olds and 1-2 per cent of 15 year olds and over wet the bed. It is however a condition which many people and their families chose to keep secret and many sufferers believe themselves to be alone.

Norgaard (1991) estimates that 10-15 per cent of all bed wetters are secondary bed wetters. In a survey of 1806 school children aged 4 to 14 years in Ireland, Devlin (1991) found the percentage of secondary bed wetters to be somewhat higher at 30 per cent. In a birth cohort study in New Zealand which followed 1265 children for the first ten years of life, Fergusson et al (1990) found that 7.9 per cent of the children had developed a secondary bed wetting problem by the age of ten years.

Bed wetting is reportedly more common in boys than girls, at least among younger children, (de Jonge, 1973; Devlin, 1991; Foxman et al 1986; Hellstrom et al, 1990; Verhulst et al, 1985), which lends some credence to those who think that bed wetting is associated with delayed physical development (Jarvelin 1989).

In a longitudinal study of untreated bed wetters Forsythe and Redmond (1974) showed an annual "spontaneous cure rate" of 14 per cent between the ages of 5 and 9 years and a 16 per cent "cure" rate between the ages of 10 and 19 years. As there is such controversy about whether bed wetting is a disease or not, it is more appropriate to say that every year the condition resolves for about one young person in six.

How frequently do individuals wet the bed?

As in many instances it is not known whether there has been one or more than one bed wetting episode in one night (because the individual often does not wake up immediately after voiding), it has become customary to use frequency of bed wetting, expressed as affected nights in a given time period (usually per week or month) as an indicator of the severity of the condition, rather than the number of episodes per night.

In their study of 1129 enuretic children, Forsythe and Redmond (1974) found that 79 per cent wet the bed seven nights per week, 11 per cent five to six nights per week and 10 per cent two to four nights per week. As the sample comprised only bed wetters attending an enuretic clinic it might be supposed that these were in the main the most severely affected children, in terms of the number of wet nights per week. Three more recent large scale epidemiological surveys, conducted in Scandinavia and Ireland by Jarvelin et al (1991), Hellstrom et al (1990) and Devlin (1991), probably give a more realistic picture of the frequency of wet nights over a given period for children living in the community, who may or may not be known to health care professionals.

From a sample of 141 children, identified as bed wetters from a survey of 3375 seven year old children in a region in Finland, Jarvelin et al (1991) found that 35 per cent wet the bed on more than 14 nights out of 30, 61 per cent wet the bed 1 to 14 nights in 30, and 5 per cent wet the bed less than once a month. In a survey of 3556 seven year old school entrants in Sweden, Hellstrom et al (1990) found a high percentage of occasional bed wetters with 64 per cent wetting less than once a week but at least once in three months.

Devlin's (1991) survey of the parents of 1806 school children aged 4 to 14 years in County Kildare, Ireland, is nearest in age range to the range of ages of the young people in this study, which was 4 to 17 years. Devlin found that 33 per cent wet the bed between once a month and less than once a week, 11 per cent wet the bed once a week, 25 per cent wet two to four nights a week, and 31 per cent wet the bed on five to seven nights a week.

What proportion of bed wetters also have day time urinary symptoms?

The prevalence of day wetting among bed wetters has been reported in several studies (e.g. Bloom et al, 1993; Blomfield and Douglas, 1956; Devlin, 1991; Fergusson et al, 1986; Hellstrom et al, 1990; Jarvelin et al, 1988 and Oppel et al, 1968a) and is estimated to be within the range of 10-20 per cent. However a comparison between studies is again made difficult because of the different definitions of day wetting used.

Hjälmås (1992) claims that 1 ml of urine is enough to cause some social inconvenience but this volume may not always be noticeable to others. Meadow (1990) has developed a three grade system which distinguishes between the loss of small and larger volumes of urine in a way which may be relevant for the young person in terms of the social consequences of incontinence and the ease or otherwise of keeping it a secret.

His grading system is:

1 Damp pants and underclothes, but urine does not seep through to the outer clothing.

2 Wetting does seep through to the trousers or skirt, making a visible wet patch.

3 A wet puddle on the seat or floor.   Meadow (1990) p.179

In his experience complete voiding in the day time (a puddle on the seat or floor) is rare. Most of the children presenting at his clinic had a mixture of Grade 1 and Grade 2 incidents.

Data on other urinary symptoms such as urgency in children is much more scarce. In a study of 3556 seven year old school entrants in Sweden, Hellstrom et al (1990) found that most children had a moderate form of urgency. Urgency was defined in Hellstrom et al's (1990, p.434) study as:

... a short latency period between first sensation and a need to void which occurred daily and was not caused by a voluntary delay.

Five per cent of the total sample were classified as having imperative urgency requiring full concentration on holding, such as assuming a squatting position.

Approaches to the management of bed wetting

This section gives an overview of approaches to the management of bed wetting from a historical perspective, from the perspective of health care professionals and from the perspective of lay people who may or may not have direct experience of caring for a bed wetting child. The purpose of this brief review is not to debate the relative merits of different treatments but to demonstrate their diversity, which may be a reflection of the lack of consensus among health care professionals on the nature of bed wetting and its aetiology.

A historical perspective

A review of treatments used in the 19th Century identified methods such as creating blisters on the sacrum, requiring a child to sleep in a frame which elevated the pelvic floor, or making young people eat porridge boiled in their own urine (Borstelmann, 1983; Buchan, 1994; Glicklich, 1951; Salmon, 1975). These would today be regarded by many as little short of child abuse, yet each method had a rational if ill-informed basis.

Health care professionals' perspective

The diversity of therapeutic approaches in common use today suggests that there is still some way to go in understanding the causes of bed wetting and the ways in which various genetic and environmental factors could be interacting. Methods in common use include:

- various forms of behavioural training (e.g. Azrin et al, 1974; Azrin & Thienes, 1978; Bollard and Nettlebeck, 1982; Butler et al, 1988, 1990; Fielding, 1980; Fordham & Meadow, 1989; Forsythe & Butler, 1989; Gustafson, 1993; Kaplan et al, 1989; Morgan, 1978; Papworth, 1989; Scott et al, 1992; van Londen et al, 1993; van Son et al, 1990; Whelan & Houts, 1990)

- pharmacologically reducing the rate and volume of urine production overnight (e.g. Hjälmås & Bengtsson, 1993; Miller et al, 1992; Rittig et al, 1989)

- pharmacologically increasing bladder capacity by diminishing detrusor contractions

- relaxation and mental imagery (e.g. Kohen, 1991)

- self hypnosis (e.g. Olness, 1975)

- visualisation (e.g. Butler, 1993a)

- hypnotherapy (e.g. Edwards & van de Spuy, 1985; Simpson, 1991)

- acupuncture (e.g. Minni et al, 1990; Xu, 1991).

Underpinning each method is a different perspective on the causes of bed wetting.

The families' perspective

As bed wetting is mostly managed by the family in the home setting, and there is some evidence that many families rarely if ever seek professional help (Devlin, 1991; Foxman et al, 1986; Haque et al, 1981) it is important to consider what parents do of their own volition to encourage the bed wetting to stop .

There is much agreement about the methods commonly used by parents as described by Bollard & Nettelbeck (1989), Butler (1987, 1994), Butler & Brewin (1986), Haque et al (1981), Morgan (1981, 1988), Shelov et al (1981) and Woolnough (1992). Many parents stop their child from taking a drink an hour or two before the young person's bed time, and lift the child at their own bed time. Many parents attribute their child's bed wetting to deep sleep and some try using an alarm clock to wake the child at a set time in the night. It is commonly reported that parents offer rewards for dry nights. Butler (1993a) and others have noted that some parents punish their children for bed wetting.

In a survey of consecutive referrals to a clinical psychologist in the UK for treatment of bed wetting, Butler et al (1993) found that only six (4.5 per cent) of the 134 mothers who completed the 20 question Maternal Tolerance Scale (Morgan and Young, 1975) answered Yes to the question: "I punish him/her for bed wetting". This is in contrast to the findings of Haque et al (1981) who found that 35.8 per cent of a total of 346 parents attending one of nine paediatric hospital departments in the United States reported on a 20 question questionnaire that they punished the child for wet nights. It is not possible to say whether the mothers in Butler et al's (1993) study under-reported the use of punishment or whether the parents define "punishment" differently in the UK and the USA, or whether there is a genuine cross-cultural difference in parents' tendency to use punishment between the UK and the USA. A comment by a health visitor tutor, quoted by Leenders (1993, p.93) suggests that it may be difficult for some parents to admit to the use of punishment:

> Corporal punishment seems no answer yet parents have 'confessed' that the bed wetting stopped after years of sympathetic understanding when the mother lost her temper and lashed out.

The impact of bed wetting on the individual and the family

This section begins with an overview of the literature on the psychological and social consequences of urinary incontinence of whatever cause, for people of all ages, before summarising what is known of the impact of bed wetting on the individual and the family.

The psychological and social consequences of urinary incontinence

Urinary incontinence has been defined by the International Continence Society Committee on Standardisation of Terminology as "involuntary loss of urine which is objectively demonstrable and a social or hygienic problem" (Abrams et al, 1988 p.17).

This definition suggests that there should be an objective assessment of the loss of urine but it also implies that incontinence is in part culturally defined and is influenced by cultural values, social norms and culturally shared rules of interpreting the event as "a social or hygienic problem".

A review of the literature from western Europe and the USA on the psychological and social effects of urinary incontinence in all age groups, whatever the cause, suggests that the involuntary loss of urine can have far reaching consequences for the individual including effects: on self-perception (Lagro-Janssen et al, 1990; Dowd, 1991; Mackaulay et al, 1991); interpersonal relationships (Parker, 1993); sexual activity (Sutherst, 1979; Norton et al, 1988) and quality of life (Herzog et al, 1988; Yu et al, 1989). Studies show that the individual's perception and interpretation of the symptoms of urinary incontinence help to determine the person's response to these symptoms, including whether or not they seek help from health care professionals (Herzog et al, 1989; Burgio et al, 1991; Rekers et al, 1992) or modify daily routines, work, leisure and social activities (Norton, 1982; Wyman et al, 1987, 1990; Hunskaar and Vinsnes, 1991).

I still have some wet nights now; usually when I get upset because I'm very lonely. I can't make friends in case they ask me to their homes, and then stay the night. I have never been away for a holiday in my life because of complaint and dare not go to cinema or any crowded place as I must dash to toilet more often than most people. So now I'm shut away in my own house, not seeing no one or having anyone to talk to and cannot make friends or join any clubs or anything. It'll hang over me to my dying day - an outcast in a modern world, always longing for a woman friend and a nice holiday.

Extract from a letter written by a 61 year old bed wetter,
cited in Stone (1973) p.1

As this quotation illustrates, bed wetting can affect some individuals into old age with devastating effects on many aspects of their lives, including the development of close personal relationships, in ways which are reminiscent of the reported effects of urinary incontinence more generally, described at the beginning of this section.

Anecdotal reports from health care professionals with a special interest in continence, such as continence nurse advisers and clinical psychologists running enuresis clinics, suggest that bed wetting can be distressing for the sufferer, of whatever age, leading to feelings of embarrassment, anxiety, loss of self esteem and occasionally physical abuse from other members of the family (Barry, 1988; Butler, 1987; Dobson, 1989; Moreton, 1989; Norton, 1986, Reinhard, 1989 and Shapiro, 1989). Sufferers are widely reported to be reluctant to stay overnight with friends, and young people are reportedly reluctant to take part in school trips which involve staying away from home (Butler, 1994). It has been suggested that bed wetting can make young people reluctant to leave home but bed wetting which persists into adulthood has also been implicated as a factor contributing to homelessness (Stone, 1973).

In her guide to enuresis for professionals, Blackwell (1989) paints a bleak picture, suggesting that persistent bed wetting may lead to: parents feeling anxious, guilty and eventually experiencing loss of confidence in their parenting skills; difficulties in the relationships between parents and children, and the child losing confidence, possibly becoming withdrawn, having difficulty making or keeping friends and under-achieving at school. Gibson (1989, p.270) describes bed wetting as "a family's recurrent nightmare" which can have devastating consequences for the family and the child's self image.

After reviewing the largely anecdotal literature on the impact of bed wetting on the individual and the family the researcher was left with three inter-related questions:

1   Are the negative and pervasive consequences of bed wetting, as reported in the literature and by the mother who triggered this study, the reality for all young people who wet the bed and their families or are they one extreme but important end of a continuum of experience?

2   Are there any bed wetters leading lives which they regard as being unaffected or only minimally affected by bed wetting?

3   Are all young people and their parents equally concerned about bed wetting?

Some light is shed on these questions by the findings of two studies.

In a study of 127 consecutive referrals to a community based enuresis clinic whose main purpose was to explore, through structured interviews, factors predicting the outcome of treatment with an enuresis alarm, Devlin and O'Cathain (1990) found that 42 per cent of parents and 32 per cent of young people were concerned "a great deal" about bed wetting, 44 per cent of parents and 34 per cent of young people rated their concern as "moderate" and 14 per cent of parents and 34 per cent of young people as "a little" or "none". This study suggests that there may be differing perceptions among young people and their parents about the impact of bed wetting on their lives but it does not answer the questions: "Who is most concerned, and why?"

In a collaborative study of parental perceptions of bed wetting involving paediatricians from nine medical centres in the United States, Haque et al (1981) found that 20 per cent of the 331 parents who completed a 20 question questionnaire were "very worried" about their child's bed wetting, 65 per cent were "concerned but not alarmed" and 14 per cent were "sometimes worried". These researchers found that parents with the least formal education were most worried about their child's bed wetting and most likely to consult a physician about it. They found that 70.6 per cent of the least educated, "Grade School", parents punished their children for bed wetting compared to 34.5 per cent of High School educated parents and 31.8 per cent of College educated parents. The Grade School parents were also found to be the most concerned about changing the wet sheets and about the smell of the wet bed. It could, however, be that the Grade School educated parents reported their feelings and practices more truthfully than the High School educated parents. There is no way of knowing from Haque's study what these parents actually did within the home, and why. The studies by Devlin and O'Cathain (1990) and Haque et al (1981) do, however, suggest that not all parents and young people are equally concerned about the bed wetting.

The family

In this section the literature on the nature of the family and the dynamics of the interaction of family members is briefly reviewed. A number of important methodological issues are raised in relation to family research.

Definitions of a "family"

> Everyone knows what a family is, yet no one seems to be able to find a definition that is acceptable to everyone. Should the definition include only those people related by blood, marriage or adoption, living under one roof ... or should a definition also include a daughter away at college, the mother's current live-in lover, the non-custodial husband and his wife, with whom the children spend every other weekend, the grandparent who lives next door but spends most of every day tending the children while the mother works ...?   Broderick (1993) p.51-52

There is no universally accepted definition of what constitutes a family (Yerby et al, 1995). Social scientists often make the distinction between the nuclear family, typically identified as a parent or parents and a child or children, and the extended family, which typically includes grandparents and other relatives. It is difficult and ultimately arbitrary to decide what is meant by a family. Definitions of the family are not widely agreed upon by families themselves (Jorgenson, 1989). Who is considered to be "family" is, in part, culturally determined. Doherty (1986) describes the family as an abstraction. Certainly there is a variety of possible definitions.

The operational definition of a family adopted at the start of this study was that it should include the young person who wet the bed and the parent or parents with whom he or she was living. This definition is compatible with the definition of a family commonly used for census purposes, which is:

> Two or more persons, sharing a common residence and related by blood, adoption or marriage   Broderick (1993) p.52

However, according to this definition a family could be two sisters living together or a married couple without children. The following more recently published definition of a family is more congruent with this study's findings,

18

encompassing as it does key concepts which facilitate an understanding of family process:

> A family is a multigenerational social system consisting of at least two interdependent people bound together by a common living space (at one time or another) and a common history, and who share some degree of emotional attachment to or involvement with one another.
>
> Yerby et al (1995) p.13

Describing a family as "multigenerational" emphasises the importance of relationships between parents and children and the influence of inter-generational influences on the family as a whole (Minuchin 1985, 1988; Simmons et al, 1993). It is the inter-gender and inter-generational nature of relationships within the family which make it unique as a social system. Unlike all other organisations families incorporate new members only by birth, adoption or marriage and members can leave only by death.

With the exception of the parent-parent dyad, relationships within families are non-voluntary. Any reorganisation of the family is generally within the control of the parents who may decide to separate, divorce and remarry irrespective of the wishes of their children. Until they are old enough to leave home young people are enmeshed as dependants in a network of relationships which may be supportive and a potent source of personal growth or which may be damaging. At the worst this unequal relationship between parents and children can lead to child abuse (Briere, 1992; Dalos and McLaughlin, 1994; Findlay and Salter, 1992; Mennen and Meadow, 1994; and Stainton-Rogers et al, 1989).

A family exerts an influence over its members which can endure for a lifetime and extend beyond one generation. It is in the family context that children first learn how valued, loved and loveable they are. Although a child's self-concept (the composite of positive and negative feelings about self) continues to grow and change throughout life, there is a growing body of evidence that many of a person's most enduring feelings about themselves are developed at an early age and are reinforced or modified by information received from other family members (e.g. Amato, 1986a,b; Belsky, 1981, 1990; Caspi and Elder, 1988; Clarke-Stewart, 1988; Cummings et al, 1989; Donley, 1993; Dunn and Brown, 1994; Eisenberg and Fabes, 1994; Gecas and Schwalbe, 1986; Hinde and Stephenson-Hinde, 1988; Lamborn et al, 1991; Noller, 1994).

Yerby et al's (1995) definition of the family given above acknowledges the family's "shared history", as well as the influence of the experiences which each parent brings to a family from their family of origin. Shared history refers

19

to the shared experiences, meanings and values associated with a family unit as it functions and evolves over time.

In Yerby et al's (1995) definition of the family, "attachment" and "involvement" refer to the intimate social bonds that link family members, which may not be visible to wider family, neighbours or researchers. "Interdependence" means that each family member's behaviour influences and is influenced by every other family member's behaviour. An acknowledgement of this characteristic of the family is pivotal to family systems theory.

Family systems theory: the family as a social system

> Study of the family in our day must include a consideration of systems theory.   Whyte (1994) p.32

The term "system" describes an integrated whole in which the parts or members are interconnected with one another in a complex web of relationships. A body of knowledge which is often referred to as family systems theory has come to form the conceptual foundation of a great deal of therapy, research and policy making in the family field (Rosenblatt, 1994).

The published works on family systems theory are so diverse (e.g. Belsky, 1981; Bronfenbrenner, 1986; Hinde, 1989; Olson, 1989; Minuchin, 1988; Patterson and Dishion, 1988) that it is misleading to write as though there is a single theory. However, the field is not chaotic. There are simply a number of perspectives such as the interpersonal perspective of Hinde or the ecological perspective of Bronfenbrenner which each focus on a different aspect of the family system and its place in the wider world.

The purpose of this overview of families as systems is to highlight common elements of these different perspectives which have helped to sensitise the researcher to the dynamics of what was going on, when analysing the data from this study. This review is also reflective, raising some fundamental methodological issues, including the extent to which a researcher can capture the reality of a situation from the family's perspective, when this reality is in a constant state of change.

In this study, family systems theory has come to be regarded as a tool for helping the researcher to see what might otherwise be missed, in the way that Rosenblatt describes:

> Thinking in terms of family systems can provide striking new realities and perspectives on what had been taken as reality; it is like being able to use microscopes and telescopes when previously one could only see things with the naked eye.   Rosenblatt (1994) p.33

Family systems theory is merely a metaphor, and like all metaphors it has both strengths and limitations. These are commented upon in Chapters 4 and 5 in relation to the extent to which the principles of family systems theory were seen to apply to the concepts which emerged during this study.

Four characteristics of the family as a system are briefly commented upon below, namely: wholeness; the inter-dependence of family members; the presence of subsystems within systems, and the dialectic between homeostasis and change.

The wholeness of the family Wholeness implies that no one element of a system can be understood in isolation from other system elements. Inherent in this concept is also the idea that the whole is more than the sum of its parts. This has important implications for any study involving the family. This stance was instinctively adopted by the researcher during the earliest phase of this study's design.

The interdependence of family members The central tenet of family systems theory is the principle of interdependent components mutually and simultaneously influencing all other system components (Broderick, 1993). The characteristic of inter-dependence is completely congruent with one of the central axioms of the naturalist paradigm, chosen to guide the selection of methods in this study, and described by Lincoln and Guba (1985) as "mutual simultaneous shaping". Yerby et al (1990, p.10) describe the general consequences of the characteristic of inter-dependence of family members:

> Inter-dependence implies that no family member is totally in control, inaccessible, or unmoved by the actions of other family members. Although one or more individuals may be accorded more power in the family unit, all individuals are affected by the actions of others.

In the second edition of their book *Understanding Family Communication* Yerby et al (1995) liken the connections between members of a family to rubber bands. Activity by one member tugs on the other members. The effect may be temporary but if the altered tension between individuals is maintained this can lead to a realignment of all family members until a new equilibrium is reached.

The concept of inter-dependence fundamentally challenges the positivist notion of linear causality (Yerby et al, 1995). Acknowledging the interdependence of family members and the principle that family members influence one another in complex and dynamic ways, encourages the researcher to move beyond the uni-directional and bi-directional approaches to understanding the interaction between parents and children which characterised most family research before 1980 (Stafford and Bayer, 1993).

The presence of subsystems within the family Minuchin (1985) describes how each family with children is composed of subsystems such as the parent-parent subsystem, and subsystems between each parent and each child and amongst siblings. In a family with two parents (P1 and P2) and two children (C1 and C2) there is the possibility of ten subsystems. While it was customary for family researchers to think in dyads such as parent-parent (P1+P2) or parent-child (eg. P1+C1), it is now acknowledged that a subsystem can develop between three members of the family which excludes the fourth, eg. P1+C1+C2 - where perhaps a step father is excluded, or P1+P2+C1, where C2 is a scapegoated child. The alliances developed between family members can have an important influence on the functioning of the family as a whole.

The response of families to change The dialectic between homeostasis and change is currently the subject of some debate between family systems theorists and is worthy of note when considering the findings of a study such as this where the emphasis is on uncovering processes and repeated patterns of behaviour. Stafford and Bayer (1993, p.31) describe the two opposing processes:

> Families resist change and strive to maintain the status quo; system members cling to current patterns of interaction. Changes are stressful, whether they are normal life-course changes or unexpected events. None-the-less, families do change. Families transform in response to each member's development as well as to the development of the constituent dyads (e.g. marital, sibling, and so forth). In addition, events that occur with the passage of time, such as the birth of a new member, an accident in the family, and so forth, modify family interaction patterns.

It is now being suggested that a family's desire to resist change has been over-stated by the earlier family systems theorists. The management of change is coming to be seen as a primary function of the family and maintenance of stability as a secondary function. Chang and Phillips (1993) have gone so far as to suggest that change is continuous and stability is an illusion.

Some phenomenologically oriented interpretivist researchers suggest that social processes are ephemeral, fluid phenomena with no existence independent of the social actors' ways of construing and describing them, so that the search for repeated patterns in behaviour is futile (Miles and Huberman, 1994). As a result of undertaking this study this researcher has

22

come to believe that patterns in parents' and young peoples' behaviour are discernible (as described in Chapters 4 and 5) but has also come to recognise the dynamic nature of reality for the family. While it is useful to be able to identify patterns in a family's interactions it is acknowledged that families are in a constant state of flux. The ability to identify stable roles and patterns of behaviour may help an understanding of a family at a point in time but as Rosenblatt (1994) points out, time and motion, like a river, keep the family in a continuous state of change.

The absence of the concept of families as systems in the literature on the management of bed wetting

While undertaking this review of the family literature in response to questions raised by the data emerging from the study, the concept of families as systems was found to be a widely accepted foundation for recent family research and to be the foundation of many therapeutic approaches to diverse family problems (Burr and Klein, 1994; Dallos, 1995; Gelles, 1995; Muncie et al, 1995; Wegner and Alexander, 1993). However, no discussion of the family as a system was encountered during the initial literature review on bed wetting suggesting that bed wetting has not been researched from this perspective.

This may be because the little research that there has been on family processes in relation to the management of bed wetting in children has been conducted by clinical psychologists. Psychologists have tended to lag behind sociologists in seeing the implications of family systems theory because, until relatively recently, the focus of psychological research has been the individual rather than the individual as part of a family group (Stafford and Bayer, 1993).

The most systematic research that there has been on family process is research led by a clinical psychologist, who has studied the consequences of "maternal intolerance" for the outcome of behavioural treatments such as the body worn alarm (Butler et al 1986, 1990, 1993), using a questionnaire originally developed by Morgan and Young (1975). The questionnaire has since been modified (Butler, 1993b; Blackwell, 1995).

In Butler's research the mother-young person dyad is the focus of interest and the research seems to be based on the premise that one aspect of a parent's personality (the attribute of maternal tolerance/intolerance) can predict the outcome of treatment for the child. This approach is sometimes referred to as the "social mould" perspective (Peterson and Rollins, 1987) whereby children are assumed to be passive and to be moulded by the actions of their parents as though they were lumps of clay. This linear, uni-directional view of the nature of parent-child interactions has long been superceded in the family literature (Stafford and Bayer, 1993).

The concept of maternal intolerance, as described by Butler, does not fully explain the wide variation in parental attitudes towards bed wetting, or their antecedents or consequences, as is made clear in Chapter 5.

Some unanswered questions

The literature review revealed that the aetiology of bed wetting is far from clear for the majority of bed wetters and is almost certainly multi-factorial. It revealed the divergence of views among health care professionals as to whether bed wetting should be categorised as pathological or not, as well as differing perspectives on how to treat it. Questions relating to the interplay between nature and nurture in this context have barely been addressed or even articulated, with many pathophysiologists dismissing the possible contribution of psychological factors to lack of night time bladder control.

A plethora of randomised controlled clinical trials of the efficacy of many different treatments was discovered. The literature also contains a number of anecdotal accounts and case histories illustrating the psychosocial consequences of bed wetting for the individual and the family. However, the review revealed a paucity of information on the ways in which bed wetting is managed within the context of everyday family life. In particular very little has been reported in the literature on the beliefs, feelings and roles of fathers and siblings.

The review confirmed that there were many unanswered questions about bed wetting and its management. It also confirmed that the phenomenon had not been widely studied from the family's perspective. The implications of these findings for the study's design are described in Chapter 2.

2 Research design and methods

Kvale (1995) argues that the quality of the knowledge produced by an investigation rests on the quality of the craftsmanship with which every stage of the research process is conducted, including: the soundness of the theoretical pre-suppositions of the study; the appropriateness of the research design and methods for the study's topic and purpose, and the rigour of the verification process. Evaluation of the craftsmanship of a study by others requires that the research procedures used be explicitly stated and transparent. This chapter briefly summarises this study's design and methods. A more detailed account of the decisions involved in designing the study and of its conduct in practice can be found in Morison (1995).

The research questions and the approach taken

> ...a researcher's reading on a subject may suggest that a new approach is needed to solve an old problem ... Something about the problem area and the phenomena associated with it remains elusive, and that something, if discovered, might be used to reconstruct understanding of this phenomenon.   Strauss and Corbin (1990) p.35

The purpose of this study, as initially envisaged, was to explore the experience and meaning of bed wetting for young people aged 5 to 20 years and their families. A review of the literature confirmed that there was a great deal still to learn about how parents manage bed wetting in the context of every day family life and its impact on everyone in the family (Chapter 1).

Prior to the first contacts with families the following broad research questions were framed:

25

1 How do parents and young people manage the practical consequences of bed wetting from day to day?

2 What impact do young people and their parents perceive bed wetting to have on the quality of their lives as individuals and on the quality of family life?

To seek answers to these questions it was decided that it would be most appropriate to use predominantly qualitative research methods, an inductive process of inquiry and grounded theory generating methods of data analysis. The paradigm guiding the approach adopted is the naturalist paradigm (Lincoln and Guba, 1985). A central axiom of the naturalist paradigm, which makes it so appropriate for the study of families as social systems (Stafford and Bayer, 1993), is the axiom of "mutual simultaneous shaping" which is the principle of interdependent components mutually and simultaneously influencing all other components. If the assumption of the interdependence of family members is accepted it becomes illogical to look for linear causality. Interactions within the family are seen as a spiral of recursive feedback loops (Minuchin, 1985). The aim becomes the search for sequenced patterns of interactions and mutual influence, which define relationships.

Data analysis began from the first contact with the first family. The following, more specific, research questions emerged during this early phase of data collection and analysis:

1 How do young people feel about wetting the bed?

2 How do parents feel about the young person's bed wetting?

3 How do families manage the day to day consequences of bed wetting?

4 What part do the different family members play in the day to day management of the young person's bed wetting?

5 What are the social consequences of bed wetting from the young person's perspective and the parents' perspective?

6 When is a young person's bed wetting identified by the family as a problem requiring action?

7 What do parents do of their own volition to encourage the young person's bed wetting to stop?

8 What are the families' experiences of the methods suggested and the help received from health care professionals?

9 What are parents' and young people's beliefs about the causes of bed wetting?

10 Where do parents' and young people's beliefs about bed wetting come from?

11 Is there a relationship between parents' beliefs about bed wetting and their behaviour towards their bed wetting child?

12 Does the young person's behaviour have any influence on the parents' behaviour in relation to the management of bed wetting?

These questions are for the most part a refinement of the broader questions initially framed, yet they rapidly took the emphasis of the study beyond a descriptive understanding of the meaning of the experience of bed wetting, from the perspective of individual family members, towards a new understanding of the processes going on within families and the conceptualisation of the family as a unique, multi-generational social system. Many more questions came to be asked of the data during analysis, in particular, questions about the relationships between emerging concepts.

Procedural implications of adopting the naturalist paradigm and a grounded theory approach

The essence of qualitative methods is induction, that is the development of theory from data. An emergent research design is axiomatic:

> N (the naturalist) elects to allow the research design to emerge (flow, cascade, unfold) rather than to construct it preordinately (*a priori*) because it is inconceivable that enough could be known ahead of time about the multiple realities to devise the design adequately.
>
> Lincoln and Guba (1985) p.41

This means starting without preconceived conceptual frameworks (Morse, 1992), making observations, identifying key concepts and patterns in the data and testing the relationships between concepts using a variety of techniques. The process is recursive. There is a purposeful grounding of the verification process in the actual data but ultimately the researcher moves beyond the data to a new understanding of the concepts pertaining to the phenomenon.

It could be argued that all naturalistic inquiry using qualitative methods which results in a theory which is grounded in the data has led to the development of a "grounded" theory. However, adopting a grounded theory approach from the outset of a study defines the generation of a theory as the primary purpose of the inquiry. The theory does not emerge as a serendipitous outcome but through the systematic use of a set of analytic procedures, as originally articulated by Glaser and Strauss (1967).

The natural setting and the family as the unit of interest The decision to conduct a study in the natural setting, which in this case was the family in the family home, acknowledges the overarching importance of the context within which the young person's bed wetting is managed from day to day. It acknowledges that something of the reality of bed wetting for the individual family members and the family as a social unit would be lost if the conversations were conducted out of context, for instance if conversations were conducted with only one family member or outwith the home.

The researcher as the principal data gathering instrument The purpose of a naturalistic inquiry is to elicit the meaning of an experience from the participant's point of view (the emic perspective) rather than from the researcher's perspective (the etic perspective). As Lincoln and Guba (1985) point out, it would be virtually impossible to devise *a priori* a non-human instrument with sufficient adaptability to encompass and adjust to the variety of realities that are likely to be encountered in the natural setting. In a naturalistic inquiry the human instrument, with all its imperfections, is the natural choice because of its adaptability and reflexivity.

Lincoln and Guba argue for the legitimation of tacit (unspoken) knowledge which may be perceived intuitively by the researcher, that is without conscious reasoning or analysis, as well as knowledge gained in language form. They suggest that the nuances of multiple realities can only be appreciated in this way. They propose that much of the interaction between the researcher and the participants occurs at an intuitive level, as it does in everyday life. External verification of the knowledge gained in this way is not possible. The inability of a conversation transcript to capture the totality of an interaction is acknowledged.

The use of supplementary data collection methods In answer to the question "Can qualitative and quantitative methods be combined?" Denzin (1978), Jick (1983), Mitchell (1986), Tripp-Reimer (1985) and Strauss and Corbin (1990) among others (who have used predominantly qualitative methods in their own

28

research) say that methods can be combined, although most research which combines methods is designed in such a way that emphasis is placed more on one approach to data collection than on the other, as in this study.

In a discussion of study design issues relating to the linking of qualitative and quantitative data, Miles and Huberman (1994) suggest that the issue is one of knowing when it is useful to count and when it is difficult or inappropriate to count at all. As Salomon (1991) points out, the issue is not a debate about the usefulness of quantitative versus qualitative methods *per se* but about whether the researcher is taking a positivist approach to understanding a few variables or a holistic approach to understanding the interaction of a multiplicity of variables in a complex environment. In their advice to researchers on designing a predominantly qualitative study, Miles and Huberman (1994, p.43) caution against falling into a "default" mode in which collecting qualitative data is seen as the only way of proceeding.

In addition to the principal data gathering method which involved in depth interviews with families, three supplementary methods of data collection were incorporated into this study's design for very specific purposes. These were:

- a urinary symptom questionnaire, completed by the family before the researcher's first visit

- diaries, in which the young person and his or her principal carer recorded events over a one month period as they actually happened and their feelings at the time

- a check list of methods used by families in the past to encourage the young person's bed wetting to stop, completed by the researcher, in consultation with the family, at the conclusion of the last visit.

Sample selection and enrolment

In quantitative research studies considerable attention is usually given to obtaining a sample which is statistically representative of the population of interest, so that generalisations may be made from the study. This is achieved through various procedures such as simple random sampling, stratified sampling, multi-stage sampling and so on.

The approach to sampling in a naturalistic inquiry is rather different from the approach adopted in many quantitative studies (where random representative sampling is used) because ultimately the sampling is on the basis of concepts that are thought to be particularly relevant to the evolving theory, rather than

29

on the basis of a few characteristics of the study participants specified in advance as being important. Sampling in qualitative research is a dynamic process in which the researcher is responsive to new concepts as they emerge. In a grounded theory study sampling continues until theoretical saturation is reached (Glaser and Strauss, 1967; Glaser, 1978). Two common approaches, which may be used in the same study and were used in this one, are selective sampling and theoretical sampling (Erlandson et al, 1993; Gilgun et al, 1992; Marshall and Rossman, 1995; Strauss and Corbin, 1990).

Selective sampling

Selective sampling precedes theoretical sampling for several reasons. The first reason is pragmatic. In order to gain access to a sample it is necessary that the research proposal be approved by an Ethics of Research Committee which usually requires a clear specification of the sample and the method of recruitment to the study. Although naturalistic inquiry requires that the researcher suspend his or her commitment to *a priori* views of the phenomenon, an investigator is highly unlikely to be without ideas about the kind of subject most likely to provide information about the phenomenon being studied. This may be because of personal or professional experience, which may have kindled an interest in the phenomenon in the first place. Ideas may also come from the review of the literature required to ensure that the knowledge being sought is not already publicly available. It is, however, important that the researcher is explicit about any preconceived ideas held at the outset of the study. The inclusion and exclusion criteria employed during initial selective sampling are given in Table 2.1.

It was decided to recruit families known to the GP or health visitor, which included one or more young people known to wet the bed, living at home with one or both parents. The age of five years was initially selected as the age from which to recruit the young people because of the consistency with which bed wetting was defined in the literature as being a problem from that age (Chapter 1). The criterion of "seven wet nights in a two week period" was used as this was the criterion proposed by Butler (1991) in his paper on the establishment of working definitions in nocturnal enuresis.

It was decided to limit the diversity of the sample by excluding young people who were wetting the bed as the result of a mental or physical illness of sufficient severity to require them to be attending a special school or to be receiving care exclusively at home. Young people living in institutionalised care, such as a children's home or boarding school were also excluded. It was, however, decided not to exclude young people where the cause of the bed wetting was known, if they were attending a normal school. The inclusion of a "deviant" case, that is one young person where the cause of the bed wetting was known for certain, proved illuminating (Chapters 4 and 5).

Table 2.1
The inclusion and exclusion criteria employed
during initial, selective sampling

Inclusion criteria	Families with one or more young people who have primary or secondary nocturnal enuresis, and who: • are aged 5 to 20 years old, and • live at home, with one or more parents, and • experience at least seven wet nights in a two week period, and • are known to the family's health visitor or general practitioner
Exclusion criteria	Families where the young person with nocturnal enuresis is sufficiently mentally or physically ill or handicapped to be: • attending a special school or day-care facilities for the mentally or physically ill or handicapped, or • receiving care exclusively at home Young people living in institutionalised care, such as a children's home or boarding school, for at least part of the time

Theoretical sampling

Theoretical sampling is sampling on the basis of concepts that have proven theoretical relevance to an evolving grounded theory, either because they are repeatedly present or notably absent when incidents are compared. The aim of theoretical sampling is to sample events rather than people *per se* to gain more understanding of: the range of conditions that give rise to the actions or inaction; how these conditions change or stay the same over time (their stability), and the consequences of these actions or inaction.

In the light of the early data analysis in this study, when it was rapidly becoming clear that many families had regarded the young person's bed wetting as a problem long before the young person had reached the age of five years old, the lower age limit for inclusion into the study was dropped and a four year old girl and her family were recruited. For similar reasons the frequency of bed wetting of "at least seven nights in a two week period" was dropped and four young people were recruited who were wetting the bed one night per week or less at the time of the study.

Recruitment continued until 19 families and 20 young people who wet the bed had been enrolled. By this time the concept of "perceived helplessness", which was thought to be the core concept, had been identified, the main categories were saturated (no new information or insights were coming to light) and the relationship between many of the concepts was becoming clear. Data analysis continued for a number of months after the last family was recruited. During this time hypotheses were constantly being compared against the data.

The enrolment process

Families thought to meet the study's initial inclusion criteria were identified by health visitors. In order that the researcher would not know the identities or addresses of families, unless they consented to take part in the study, the researcher gave the health visitor: a recently dated but non-personalised letter explaining the nature of the study and its purpose; a consent form, to be completed by parents and the young person if aged 16 years or over, if they agreed to take part, and a stamped envelope, addressed to the researcher at the researcher's academic institution. These were contained in a blank envelope which the health visitor was asked to address. The health visitor then decided whether to post the letter to the family or to deliver it by hand at her next visit. This mechanism was decided upon by the health visitors themselves. In total 51 per cent of families identified by health visitors and who were sent or given the letter about the study, agreed to take part.

Data collection

The nature of the involvement of families is illustrated in Figure 2.1.

32

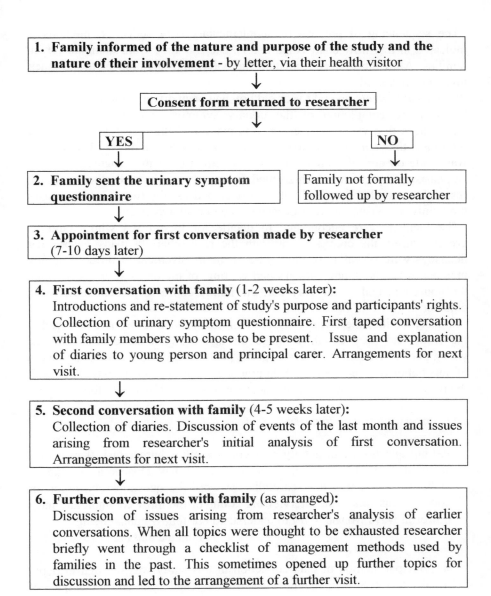

1. **Family informed of the nature and purpose of the study and the nature of their involvement** - by letter, via their health visitor

↓

Consent form returned to researcher

↓

YES   NO

↓   ↓

2. **Family sent the urinary symptom questionnaire**

Family not formally followed up by researcher

↓

3. **Appointment for first conversation made by researcher** (7-10 days later)

↓

4. **First conversation with family** (1-2 weeks later):
Introductions and re-statement of study's purpose and participants' rights. Collection of urinary symptom questionnaire. First taped conversation with family members who chose to be present. Issue and explanation of diaries to young person and principal carer. Arrangements for next visit.

↓

5. **Second conversation with family** (4-5 weeks later):
Collection of diaries. Discussion of events of the last month and issues arising from researcher's initial analysis of first conversation. Arrangements for next visit.

↓

6. **Further conversations with family** (as arranged):
Discussion of issues arising from researcher's analysis of earlier conversations. When all topics were thought to be exhausted researcher briefly went through a checklist of management methods used by families in the past. This sometimes opened up further topics for discussion and led to the arrangement of a further visit.

Figure 2.1   **The nature of the involvement of families**

33

The sequencing of the use of supplementary data collection methods is indicated in this flow chart (Figure 2.1). Steps 1 to 4 were common for all families. After the first conversation the nature and duration of the families' involvement varied.

In one case, where an eight year old boy had been dry at night for two weeks between the completion of the urinary symptom questionnaire and the researcher's first visit, the decision was made that the researcher would not return and the young person would not be asked to keep a diary. This decision was made on ethical grounds for fear of setting back the progress made by emphasising a problem which seemed to have resolved. In all other cases the researcher revisited the family at least once and usually twice. In three cases the family was visited on four occasions, by mutual agreement.

The families were encouraged to decide for themselves who would be present during the conversations with the researcher. In many cases their decisions were revealing of the nature of the involvement of different family members with the young person's bed wetting, of the division of tasks within the household and of the way that the family chose to present itself to an outsider.

In many families there was evidence that the decision to become involved in the study had been carefully talked through between the parents and the young person. Obtaining access to participants involved a continuous process of negotiation and re-negotiation. In practice the arrangements associated with the researcher's visits were for the most part controlled by the mothers.

The conversations with families

> Asking questions and getting answers is a much harder task than it may seem at first. The spoken or written word has always a residue of ambiguity, no matter how carefully we word the questions and report or code the answers. Yet, interviewing is one of the most common and most powerful ways we use to try to understand our fellow human beings.
>
> Fontana and Frey (1994) p.361

The principal method of data collection in this study was through in depth informal interviews with families. The special challenges and techniques of informal, in depth interviewing have been described in detail in many articles and texts on research methods, such as Barker (1991), Chenitz (1986), Fielding (1993), Fontana and Frey (1994), Gilgun et al (1992), Gray (1994), Jones (1985), May (1991), Oppenheim (1992) and Rose (1994). There is not the space here to dwell on all of the issues raised in these books and articles. Instead attention is given to some issues of particular relevance to this study, such as the communication skills which may be brought to conversations with families by a nurse, the special challenges of interviewing children and adolescents, the challenges posed by the presence of younger children and the researcher's relationship with families as a fellow human being.

Some consequences of the principal data gatherer being a nurse Many of the skills required for conducting in depth interviews such as: building rapport; active listening; open-ended questioning; restating and seeking clarification; focusing and summarising and paying close attention to non-verbal communication are also the skills required for effective communication in nursing practice, as described for example by Burnand (1989), Coutts and Hardy (1985), Ewles and Simnett (1992), Heron (1991), Porritt (1990) and Tschudin (1991). A nurse may well come to a research study with well developed inter-personal communication skills which are of pivotal importance when communicating with research participants.

Chenitz (1986, p.85) describes another advantage of being a nurse:

The nurse image can be very useful to gain the confidence of informants. People identify nurses with a caring, nurturing role. Further, people will talk to nurses and reveal to them content that they may not be so willing to disclose to others.

There are, however, heavy responsibilities and ethical issues relating to the researcher who is known to be a nurse, of which perhaps the most central is the participants' expectation that the researcher will intervene in a clinical role should this be needed (Chenitz, 1986; Dunn, 1991; Wilde, 1992). It was for this reason that the researcher discussed her non-clinical role with the families at the outset and always referred the family back to the health visitor for specific advice, when this was sought. This position was readily accepted by the families who, for the most part, seemed glad to have the opportunity to discuss their feelings with someone who was not directly involved with their care.

The particular challenges of conversations with children and adolescents In the past researchers have relied almost exclusively on adults (usually parents or teachers) as the primary informants for data concerning children's thoughts and feelings (Broderick, 1993; Deatrick and Faux, 1991; Faux et al, 1988; Stafford and Bayer, 1993):

The traditional socialization and developmental perspectives view children as being unable to describe and understand their world and life experiences due to developmental immaturity (cognitive and linguistic) and to a lack of socialization experiences.   Deatrick and Faux (1991) p.203

However there are those, such as Amato and Ochiltree (1987) who view children as competent interpreters of their world:

Overall, our data suggests that if researchers stick to the here-and-now they can achieve articulate and informative responses from children about their families.   Amato and Ochiltree (1987) p.674

It is important, however, to recognise the limits imposed by children's cognitive, social and linguistic skills, which vary enormously along the developmental life span as well as between individuals (Hetherington and Parke, 1993; Mussen et al, 1990).

The ability of the researcher to gain the trust of the young person and the researcher's range of interpersonal skills are, if anything, even more important when conducting research involving children than in research involving adults. This is especially the case when talking with the youngest children whose linguistic and social skills are likely to be least developed and who are most likely to exhibit anxiety of strangers. The researcher needs to be flexible and inventive and to have a sufficient understanding of children's developmental stage and language levels to stand any chance of entering into the child's world, even to a limited extent.

When conversing with the young people in this study time was spent in getting to know them, after a simple introduction of the researcher as a nurse who was doing a "project" about bed wetting. The idea of research as a "project" was explored in relation to projects that the young people were involved in at school, to facilitate the young person's understanding that a project was about "finding out more about something, which might be helpful to know". The researcher's status as a nurse may well have legitimised the inquiry in the young people's eyes, as well as in the parents' eyes.

To facilitate an exploration of feelings, many of the young people were asked to draw pictures of themselves in concrete situations such as on waking up to find the bed wet. They were then asked to tell the researcher about the picture, to help remove any ambiguity and to encourage the young person to share his or her feelings. The sensitivity of the topic was to some extent anticipated. It showed itself most clearly in non-verbal behaviour.

To overcome linguistic barriers, especially for the very young children, cards were made of the faces scale developed by Andrews and Withey (cited in

McDowell and Newell, 1987 p.215). This scale was used by Anderson and Bury (1988) to gain insights into people's feelings about life 18 months after a stroke. In the present study the purpose of using the cards was to help the young people to explore feelings for which they might not have the words. The young people were asked what the faces signified to them and their responses were interpreted accordingly. The meaning of the middle face is ambiguous. Some of the older children described it as being "between happy and sad", some as "no feelings", some as "grumpy".

In practice, many young people, who were very shy about talking about their bed wetting, were able to communicate graphically what their feelings were with the help of the cards and to indicate their perception of the feelings of other members of the household, in a way which showed that they were able to make fine discriminations (Morison, 1995). The cards were merely used to facilitate communication. Sometimes only one card was used. Many of the children regarded the cards as a game which they greatly enjoyed:

MOYA: How do you feel about taking part in this project?
JOHN: Happy.
MOYA: Why that one? [he has ticked a very happy face on a "faces-feelings" card].
JOHN: Well, it's the first time I've ever been in a project with adults and that and I'm really happy. I've not done a project like this before. It's really good. I'm enjoying myself.
MOYA: What was the best thing?
JOHN: Doing the faces and the pictures.   John (age 8)

It is extremely difficult for an adult not to be in control of an interaction with a child yet the young people were encouraged from the outset to determine the agenda. To postpone talking about bed wetting, and to show the researcher what he could do, John, quoted above, had systematically emptied the contents of his school bag, reading a story that he had written, reading from his evening's reading assignment from school and reciting a hymn that he was learning for Easter.

Any leads given by the children were followed up, but sometimes a straight question such as: "Tell me about the bed wetting", which could lead to an illuminating response from a parent, and indicate areas of special concern, would lead to no more than a shrug of the young person's shoulders, which was in itself revealing.

The challenges posed by the presence of younger children On a number of occasions the mothers decided to speak with the researcher before the young person returned from school. In many of these cases the mother was looking after other younger children at the time. This posed special challenges to the researcher's inter-personal and interviewing skills.

In four families in particular, where the mother was looking after one or more children under school age, the researcher found herself in the dual position of being both interviewer and child minder, entertaining up to three other children with the help of coloured paper and pens, while attempting to talk with the young person who wet the bed. At these times the researcher had the feeling that she had truly entered into the family's rather chaotic world. Or perhaps it was that some of these mothers were happy to take the opportunity to sit quietly for a few moments while someone else entertained the children. The tranquillity achieved by the researcher as four toddlers were absorbed with their drawing was described by one, usually distracted mother as: "no' normal!"

The researcher as more than a human data gathering instrument The conversations with both the children and their parents required patience and adaptability. Above all they required empathy and unconditional acceptance of all the family members, which is also, ultimately, the basis of any therapeutic intervention (Tschudin, 1991).

The children and their parents reciprocated in so many ways, most of all by sharing their experiences and feelings with the researcher over several occasions. Some of the children gave the researcher small gifts which they had made. One of the most touching gifts was a thank you card from one family signed: "from all of us".

The mother of the family who seemed the most uncomfortable about taking part in this study unexpectedly sent a note, eight months later, enclosing some diary forms that she had come across:

Dear Moya,
May I take this opportunity in thanking you for helping with the bed wetting problem. Paul has been dry since the autumn, already it seems a long time ago and one forgets the past routines ... Your help did stop us getting bogged down in the problem.

Although every effort was made to minimise any potentially adverse effects for the young people and their families of participating in this study, there was no secondary therapeutic agenda and the families were referred back to their health visitor for specific advice. Talking about the situation openly within the family may, however, have led family members to review their beliefs, feelings and behaviour towards one another.

The use of computer software to facilitate data storage and data handling

In their book *Basics of qualitative research: grounded theory procedures and techniques*, which formed an invaluable and much used guide during the analysis of data in this study, Strauss and Corbin (1990) barely mention the use of computer software to facilitate data storage, handling and analysis. It is easy to understand, on an intuitive level, why some researchers feel that the use of computer software could stifle the creativity of the processes involved in inductive analysis. There is also the largely unspoken fear that a computer is like a genie in a bottle which, once released, will transform the activity of field research in unnoticed and unwelcome ways (Lee and Fielding, 1993).

In an article entitled "The right brain strikes back" Agar (1993) describes the dangers of what he calls "computer lust" (p.182) where the means become the end. In what he calls his paranoid fantasy he sees computers mutating from an item in a context to the context itself. The main counter to this argument is that the fault lies not with the computer software but with the researcher who uses it inappropriately.

Becker (1993) suggests that the use of computers for data analysis in grounded theory studies results in flat and over simplified descriptive results. If the software were effectively left to itself this could conceivably happen but the use of computer software to facilitate theory generation and testing does not replace the right brain's ability to make conceptual connections from data from social situations that appear at first to be quite different. Instead, by facilitating and greatly speeding up the clerical tasks associated with data handling, it can free up the researcher's time (Tesch, 1990, 1991) to discover theory creatively and intuitively in the way that Glaser and Strauss (1967) originally conceived it.

The final decision to use a computer software package to aid data storage, data handling and some aspects of data analysis was taken after a careful analysis of the nature of the task in hand and an appraisal of the facilities provided by the software then available. With the stated and over-arching purpose of theory building in mind, the following facilities were sought:

- a flexible coding system into which new codes could be added at any time

- powerful search facilities

- a theory testing capability

- a way of keeping track of the project.

A search of the literature on the use of computers in qualitative research uncovered articles and books by among others: Anderson (1987); Huber and Garcia (1991); Knafl and Webster (1988); Morse (1991b); Pfaffenberger (1988); Richards and Richards (1991); Russell and Gregory (1993) and Tesch (1991). The most useful books on the subject were found to be Fielding and Lee's (1993) book *Using computers in qualitative research* and Tesch's (1990) book *Qualitative analysis: analysis types and software tools.*

Almost any article or book on computer software is likely to be out of date in many aspects of detail before it is published as the field is moving forward so quickly. In an attempt to make a decision based on the most up to date information the major suppliers of software suitable for qualitative research were contacted for the latest information about their products.

With this study's emphasis on theory building rather than description, the NUD•IST package was finally selected because of the power of its hierarchical indexing system. NUD•IST stands for Non-numerical Unstructured Data: Indexing, Searching and Theorising. One reason why NUD•IST appeared from the outset to be and has proved to be so appropriate for this study is that it was designed by Tom Richards for his wife Lynn, who has extensive experience of grounded theory methods of analysis and of conducting research with families.

Since the decision was taken to use NUD•IST there have been many valuable additions to the literature on the use of computers as an aid to qualitative research analysis. An article by Richards and Richards (1994a) gives a comprehensive exposition on the issues relating to the use of computers to facilitate a wide range of qualitative research approaches. Weitzman and Miles' (1995) book *Computer programmes for qualitative data analysis* is another authoritative text. Ultimately a researcher's decision to use a computer programme to facilitate data handling and data analysis is a personal one and needs to be based on a thorough understanding of the purpose of the inquiry and an appraisal of the facilities of the different packages available at the time.

The use of a computer software package can shift the balance of time spent on the mechanics of data handling *per se* and on data analysis, strongly in favour of data analysis, by considerably speeding up the clerical tasks involved in searching for and retrieving data. Gerson (1984) suggests that the principal benefit of computer technology is its potential for increased rigour in analysis. Freeing up time and energy for the researcher to think creatively is perhaps one of the most compelling reasons for using computer software, especially when the time so spent leads to the development of a powerful, precise and tightly integrated theory. The ways in which NUD•IST has been used in practice are briefly described and demonstrated below.

Inductive data analysis

Induction is the essence of naturalistic inquiry and the basis of the grounded theory approach to data analysis. Induction involves the development of theory from data. Concepts are ultimately the units of interest in grounded theory research. All the procedures described in this section have the purpose of identifying, developing and relating concepts. The analytic process is recursive. There is a constant interplay between proposing and checking. This is what makes the theory developed "grounded" in the data. An interactive model of the components of data analysis is given in Figure 2.2.

Before describing some of the analytic procedures used in this study a personal quality required of the researcher is described, which is central to the process of inductive analysis. The quality is sometimes referred to as "theoretical sensitivity" (Glaser, 1978), and is described by Strauss and Corbin (1990, p.42) in the following terms:

> Theoretical sensitivity refers to the attribute of having insight, the ability to give meaning to data, the capacity to understand, and capability to separate the pertinent from that which isn't. All this is done in conceptual rather than concrete terms.

Theoretical sensitivity is a requirement for the creativity which can help to uncover new ways of looking at a phenomenon. It comes from a number of sources. These include a knowledge of the literature and the professional and personal experience of the researcher. These are the background that the researcher brings to the situation. Theoretical sensitivity can also be acquired through the analytic process itself. Insight and understanding increase as the researcher interacts with the data. Regarding all categories, explanations and tentative theories as provisional until convincingly supported by data, and following the coding procedures outlined below, has helped to give rigour to this study.

Open coding and the use of memos and diagrams

Open coding is the process of breaking down, examining, comparing, conceptualising and categorising data. The processes involved in open coding are described by Corbin (1986), Miles and Huberman (1994) and others. The purpose is to identify and name phenomena, which is a necessary first step in concept development. From the time of the earliest analysis of the first conversations with families the emerging categories were identified and named. The coding was refined and new codes added in an ongoing way.

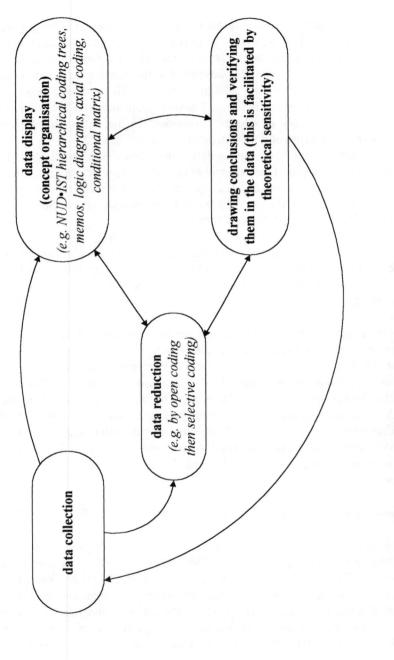

Figure 2.2   An interactive model of the components of data analysis
(Modified from Miles and Huberman (1994) p.12)

Keeping a track of the coding was at first achieved by updating a loose leaf coding book with the aid of a word processing package. Six months into the study this tedious process was transformed with the help of the NUD•IST software package.

Two analytic procedures which help with concept clarification are making comparisons and asking questions. These procedures were used constantly. This is what is meant when a grounded theory approach is described as a "constant comparative" method of inquiry (Glaser and Strauss, 1967). Memos and diagrams were used as adjunctive procedures throughout the eighteen months of data analysis to help to explore the possible relationships between concepts, using techniques described by Glaser (1978); Corbin (1986); Miles and Huberman (1994) and Richards and Richards (1991, 1994b).

Developing a hierarchical indexing system

Richards and Richards (1994b) liken NUD•IST's indexing system to a library index which enables the researcher to store and locate data very easily. If the indexing (coding) categories are organised hierarchically the result is an indexing tree which is like a map of the project. Each node on the tree is like a pigeon-hole in which "like" data and the researcher's thoughts about them can be stored. The software has been designed to enable the indexing system to grow and change shape as the researcher's thinking about a project grows and develops. At any point in time it shows the concepts being explored and it is therefore a reflection of the progress of the researcher's analytical thinking. Over a one year period a hierarchical indexing system was developed to store the researcher's thinking about the study. The sequence of the steps involved in data transcription, importing, coding, search and retrieval is illustrated in Figure 2.3.

Lynn Richards regards the development of the indexing system and the coding (indexing) of data as much more than just a clerical exercise:

> Decisions are being made about what is a category of significance to the study, what questions are being asked, what concepts developed, what ideas explored, and whether these categories should be altered, re-defined, or deleted during analysis.   Richards and Richards (1994a) p.447

The way in which a small part of the indexing system was developed is described below to illustrate the analytic processes involved.

Figure 2.4 illustrates part of the indexing system which emerged from mothers' comments on their beliefs about various aspects of the young person's bed wetting.

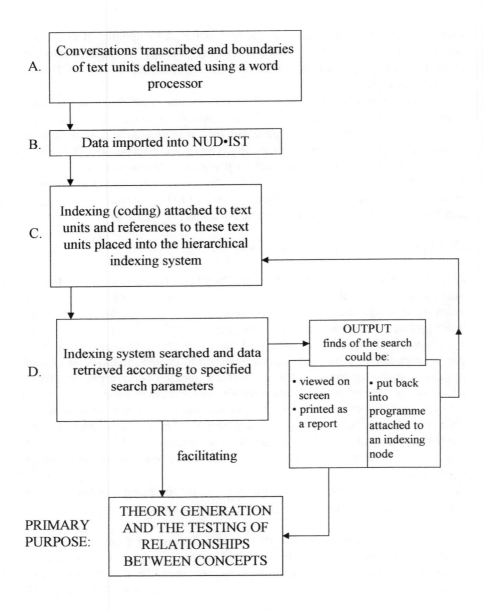

Figure 2.3   A flow diagram of the processes of data transcription, importing, coding, searching and retrieval using the computer software package: NUD•IST Power Version 3.0

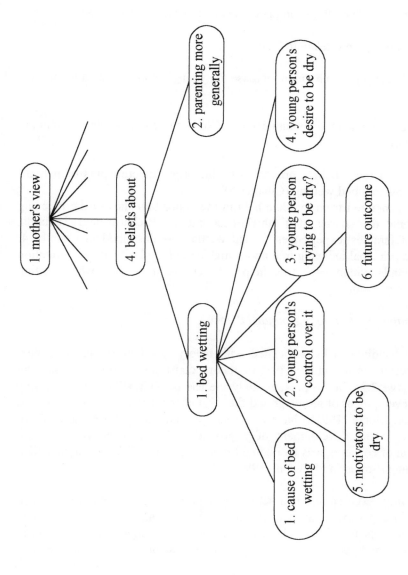

Figure 2.4 Part of the indexing system for mothers' beliefs about bed wetting and parenting more generally

The six sub-categories which emerged during conversations with mothers as important to them were the mothers' perceptions of:

1 the cause of the bed wetting

2 the young person's control over the phenomenon

3 the extent to which the young person was making an effort to be dry

4 the young person's desire to be dry

5 possible factors which might increase the young person's motivation to be dry, and

6 whether and when the young person would become reliably dry at night in the future.

The nature of these beliefs proved to be important determinants of parents' attitudes towards bed wetting (Chapter 5).

Reports generated from the data held in the major branches of the indexing tree became the source of a "thick description" (Richards and Richards, 1994a) of families' experiences of bed wetting, as described in Chapter 4. While the principal indexing tree nodes highlighted the broad issues, attention to the details within each tree helped to ensure a balance when writing descriptive accounts.

Constructing and testing a grounded theory

The data handling tasks associated with theory development are complex. Theory testing is an integral part of theory construction, not a subsequent stage (Figure 2.2). In the present study the use of NUD•IST paved the way for the development of an integrated theory. Other researchers such as Dowd (1991) and Morse (1991b) have also found a computer programme to be of assistance in the development of a grounded theory. However the final integration of concepts was facilitated by the use of a coding paradigm, called axial coding (Strauss and Corbin, 1990).

Axial coding Axial coding is a set of procedures whereby data are put back together in a new way, after open coding, by making connections between categories. This is achieved by using a coding paradigm involving: causal conditions (conditions which give rise to a phenomenon); the phenomenon or central idea; aspects of the context in which the phenomenon is embedded; intervening conditions; action/interactional strategies; and the consequences or outcomes of action and interaction. The linking and development of categories takes place with the help of the basic analytical procedures used from the very outset of open coding such as asking questions about what is going on, when and why, and making comparisons of instances of the phenomenon to gain an understanding of the conditions in which events take place.

The process of axial coding is quite complex because the analysis involves performing four distinct analytic steps almost simultaneously. These are:

1   the hypothetical linking of concepts

2   the verification of the hypotheses against data

3   the continued search for the properties of the concepts and their dimensions, and

4   an exploration of the variation in expression of the phenomenon.

This involves moving back and forth between inductive and deductive thinking.

The identification of the core concept The identification of what was initially believed to be the core concept of "perceived helplessness" occurred in the earliest stages of open coding. It was used to code the second line of the first transcript of the first conversation with the first family to be enrolled into the study and it returned in many guises later on. However the central phenomenon around which all the other categories were integrated became apparent during the later stages of analysis and was found to be "perceived control", as is described in Chapter 5, which usually manifested as perceived helplessness.

Ethical issues

This section briefly highlights some ethical issues relating to research involving young people who wet the bed. A more detailed discussion of issues of universal concern for research involving human subjects such as informed consent, privacy, confidentiality and data protection and issues relating to family research, as they pertained to this study, is given in Morison (1995).

Suspected child abuse

The possibility of encountering child abuse was anticipated. Mechanisms for referral in the case of suspected child abuse were discussed with clinicians during the consultation phase of this study. The Region's Inter-Agency Procedural Guidelines were adopted. Only one case of child abuse was knowingly encountered. The abuse had occurred in the past and at the time of the study the perpetrator had been in prison for the offence for 18 months.

Discovering an unmet medical need

The other issue anticipated in advance of meeting with the families was discovering an unmet need for medical care. Criteria for referring a family back to their GP for further assessment of urinary continence problems were discussed with some of the families' GPs and with a senior consultant urologist. It was jointly decided that specific referral criteria would be haematuria or a suspected urinary tract infection. It was agreed that requests for further information about the management of bed wetting or any other clinical issue would be passed back to the health visitor, in the first instance, with the family's consent.

Raising the spectre of a problem with no ending

Both ethical and theoretical considerations influenced the decisions taken during the process of data gathering to pursue some lines of inquiry and not others. It was quickly recognised that many parents and young people had come to regard the bed wetting as a never ending problem and had come to believe themselves to be helpless to influence the situation. In a few instances parents and young people expressed feelings of both helplessness and hopelessness. Great care was taken not to raise the spectre of the possible long term nature of the bed wetting within those families where this issue had not spontaneously emerged.

3 An introduction to the families

In this study the family is seen both as the context in which a young person's bed wetting is managed and as a unit of interest in its own right. The focus of interest and the units of data collection and data analysis therefore encompass both individuals within the family and the family as a whole social unit, which in turn is seen as being embedded within a local community, set in a wider society (Figure 3.1).

As is described in Chapter 1, there are many perspectives on the family among family systems theorists. Some, such as Bronfenbrenner (1986), take an ecological perspective, choosing to focus on the family within the context of the wider social systems of community and society. Other researchers, such as Hinde (1989), are more concerned with the nature and dynamics of interpersonal relationships within the family. In the present study the focus has been on the conditions affecting the action and interaction of family members and the consequences of these actions for the individuals involved and the family as a social unit. Some of the conditions identified have been at the ecological level and some at the individual level. The processes studied have for the most part been at the relational and interactional level, that is between members of a family living within the same household.

Up until now the phenomenon of bed wetting has mostly been researched at the individual, pathophysiological, organ system level, that is at the level of bladder function. In the few studies where a more family oriented approach has been taken, the research has been conducted at the level of the mother-child sub-system, based on a unidirectional conceptualisation of the nature of the parent-child relationship (Chapter 1). In the present study a new approach has been taken to understanding a common condition of childhood, by focusing on the impact of bed wetting on the family as a social system.

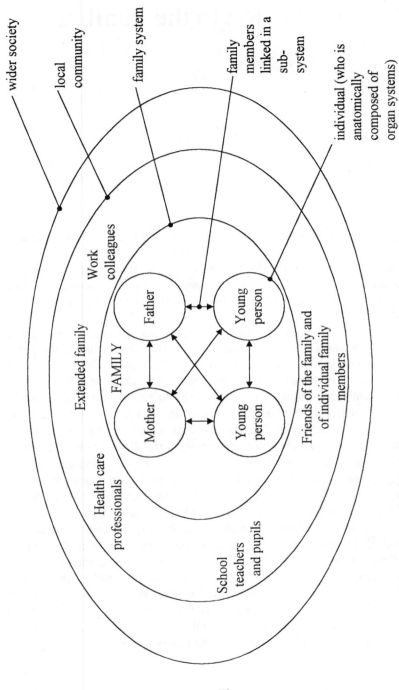

Figure 3.1 The conceptualisation of the family as a system, embedded within systems and composed of sub-systems

The aim has been to take a holistic approach to understanding the interaction of a multiplicity of variables on many system levels. While the focus of this study is predominantly at the level of the family, there are many hints that society's view of bed wetting and the attitude of extended family, friends, and health care professionals in the local community, have an impact on the family's experience of bed wetting, as does the nature of the young person's urinary symptoms. Failure to acknowledge the actual or potential impact of influences at these system levels on the family's experience of bed wetting would be both parochial and short-sighted.

This chapter sets the scene for the chapters that follow by summarising certain contextual data at the local community, family and individual levels.

The study area

This study was conducted within an area of central Scotland served by Forth Valley Health Board. The sample of 19 families was drawn from 11 GP practices. Four of the families live in a rural ward in West Stirlingshire. The other 15 families live within five miles of Stirling town centre.

In Forth Valley there are neither the concentrations of deprivation nor of male unemployment that are to be found in other areas of Scotland such as Greater Glasgow. Male unemployment in Forth Valley was 11.9 per cent in 1991, (approximately mid way between Greater Glasgow at 20.6 per cent and the Shetland Islands at 5.6 per cent) ranging from 4 to 32 per cent locally by electoral ward.

Analysis of census-based deprivation indices for the district council electoral wards in which the families lived, undertaken after data collection was completed, confirmed the researcher's local knowledge that the families came from a wide spectrum of communities, from the relatively affluent to amongst the most deprived in the area. Six of the 19 families were drawn from three of the five wards assessed as having the greatest deprivation in the whole of Forth Valley. By contrast 3 of the 19 families came from two of the five most affluent wards.

The families

The young people

The twenty young people enrolled into this study ranged in age from 4 to 17 years with a mean age of 10. There were 12 males and 8 females. In one family the bed wetters were twins. All the young people were still attending school, the youngest was attending nursery school.

With one exception, the cause of the young person's bed wetting was not known. The exception was Michael (age 8), who has congenital bladder neck obstruction and only one, partially functioning kidney. He is in chronic renal failure and his symptoms include polyuria (the production of large volumes of dilute urine). The inclusion of Michael has proved a valuable case for comparison with the majority of cases where the cause of the bed wetting has not been identified.

Family composition

Each of the 19 families enrolled into this study included a young person known locally to the health visitor to wet the bed, and his or her natural mother. Three families were headed by a lone mother who was separated or divorced from the young person's natural father. The remaining households included the young person's natural father, a stepfather, or the mother's current male partner. Four of the young people currently had two father figures in their lives, their natural father with whom they stayed on occasions and a stepfather or the mother's male partner with whom they lived for most of the time.

The relationship of the parents in each family at the time of the study and the number of times that the families had been re-ordered is summarised in Appendix A. Re-ordering refers to the number of times that the parental composition of the household had changed within the young person's lifetime. In all, over half the young people in this study had experienced some form of family re-organisation. The literature suggests that family re-organisation associated with divorce and re-marriage has become an increasingly common experience in the lives of parents and children (Hetherington, 1992). There is growing evidence that divorce and re-marriage pose adaptive challenges to family members and involve alterations in family functioning; however, the short and long term effects of family transitions are far from clear cut.

In the present study one lone mother was finding it particularly difficult to cope with caring for her four children and described her relationship with her bed wetting daughter as poor. However the other two lone mothers and the six mothers who had re-married, or had entered into a relationship with a new male partner, appeared to have found a new stability in their lives and five of them described their relationships with their children as good.

For two of the families in this study, which comprised both of the young person's natural parents, tension between the parents was reported by the mothers to be high and both mothers reported behavioural problems in their

52

children. Many family theorists view the quality of the marital relationship and the couple's satisfaction with it as having all-important effects on other family relationships (Amato, 1986a; Belsky et al, 1991; Grych and Fincham, 1990).

The effects of the young person's bed wetting on relationships within the family are discussed in Chapter 4. One father was said by the mother to have threatened to leave the family because of it. It is not, however, possible to say whether a young person's bed wetting merely exacerbates problems between family members, where relationships are already poor, or whether the bed wetting is a primary cause of the problem.

Parents' personal history of bed wetting

It was discovered in conversation that six mothers had themselves been bed wetters. Four mothers who had not wet the bed themselves had had a bed wetting sibling and had had some responsibility for their sibling's care. The natural fathers of four of the young people were said by their wives to have wet the bed (Appendix A).

There is evidence to suggest that there is a genetic component to the aetiology of bed wetting (Eiberg et al, 1995). Bakwin (1973) found that where both parents had been bed wetters 77 per cent of their children were bed wetters, and if one of the parents had wet the bed 44 per cent of their children experienced the problem. In Bakwin's study where neither of the parents had been a bed wetter, only 15 per cent of their children were affected.

In this study there was found to be a strong relationship between the nature of parents' previous experiences of bed wetting and their feelings, attitudes, and behaviour towards their own bed wetting child (Chapters 4 and 5).

The night and day time urinary symptoms of the young people who wet the bed

In this section the young people's night and day time urinary symptoms are described, based on an analysis of data from the urinary symptom questionnaire completed by the young people and their parents before the researcher's first visit and an analysis of the conversations with families.

The frequency of bed wetting

The frequency of the young people's bed wetting, expressed as wet nights per week, is given in Table 3.1. Four of the young people were said to be wetting the bed on one night per week or less. Five were wetting the bed 2 to 4 nights per week and 11 were wetting the bed 5 to 7 nights per week. These findings are broadly in line with the findings of several surveys of the frequency of bed wetting in young people (Chapter 1).

A dimension of bed wetting, that neither the urinary symptom questionnaire nor epidemiological surveys highlight is the way in which the frequency of bed wetting can fluctuate widely for some individuals over time. The fluctuating nature of the frequency of bed wetting became apparent during conversations with families. For many young people the number of wet nights per week was said to have reduced, at first, with treatment but in most cases the young person's progress had not been maintained.

Table 3.1
Frequency of bed wetting (nights per week)*

Nights per week	Male	Female	Total	% of total
7	3	4	7	35
6	2	1	3	15
5	-	1	1	5
4	-	1	1	5
3	3	-	3	15
2	1	-	1	5
1 or less	3	1	4	20

* source of data is urinary symptom questionnaire

In some cases the parents had their own "theory" to account for setbacks. Some mothers associated the increase in the number of wet nights with events occurring within the family at the time (Chapter 5). In most cases, however, both young people and their parents were puzzled when progress was not maintained.

It became apparent that four inter-related aspects of the frequency of bed wetting affected individuals' feelings about it, namely:

54

- the proportion of "wet" nights in the week (constancy)

- whether the frequency of dry nights was increasing, static or decreasing (presence or absence of progress)

- the extent to which the frequency of bed wetting and any changes in its frequency could be accounted for (predictability)

- the individual's perception of his/her ability to influence progress in a positive way (controllability).

Parents' and young people's beliefs about the causes of bed wetting and their control over it are discussed in Chapter 5. The constancy of some young people's bed wetting and its uncontrollability had caused many young people and their parents to feel helpless and despairing at some point and for some individuals these were the predominant feelings at the time of the study.

Primary and secondary bed wetting

Norgaard (1991) estimates that 10 to 15 per cent of bed wetters are secondary bed wetters. Three boys in the present study, where the cause of the bed wetting was not known, were initially classified as secondary bed wetters (Table 3.2), using Hjälmås (1992, p.5) definition of secondary childhood incontinence which is "a child who has been dry for a period of at least six months and then starts to wet again".

These three boys were said by their parents to have been reliably dry for between one and two years before recommencing bed wetting at the ages of 3½ to 4 years. According to some definitions these boys would not have been classified as secondary bed wetters at all, although they had been reliably dry for so long, as they had re-started bed wetting before the age of five. The failure to classify children who have been dry for one to two years as secondary bed wetters could have implications for randomised controlled trials conducted in young people who are all supposedly primary bed wetters.

The mothers clearly remembered the circumstances in which the bed wetting had recommenced. In the case of the twins, Stephen and John (age 8), the bed wetting had started shortly after the parents had separated and the twins had entered a homeless unit with their mother. Stephen was said to have been particularly badly affected by the experience and at the time of this study, four years later, he was still wetting the bed seven nights per week. John's bed wetting had considerably improved over the intervening years and by the time of the study he was only wetting the bed three nights per week.

Table 3.2
Frequency of primary and secondary bed wetting*

	Male	Female	Total	% of total
Primary bed wetting				
a. never totally dry at night	7	4	11	55
b. reliably dry at night but for less than six months	1	3	4	20
c. not known if ever dry at night	-	1	1	5
Secondary bed wetting	3	-	3	15
Cause known (congenital bladder neck obstruction, only one partially functioning kidney and chronic renal failure)	1	-	1	5

* sources of data are urinary symptom questionnaire and conversations with parents

The mother of Gary (age 5) linked the re-commencement of her son's bed wetting to the natural father coming to live in the family home. She said that she and her son had been happily living with her parents before that time and Gary had been out of nappies and reliably dry for a year. The onset of the secondary incontinence was also said to have been very sudden.

An observation which emerged through conversations with parents in the study, but not from the urinary symptom questionnaire (which asked whether the young person had ever had a period of at least 6 months when they had been dry every night), was that four of the "primary" enuretics had been out of nappies at night and had been reliably dry for several months, but less than six months, when the bed wetting had suddenly recommenced (Table 3.2).

In three of these cases the young person was quite clearly described as being emotionally upset when the bed wetting recommenced. In one case the young person's father had died. In another case the circumstances surrounding the re-commencement of the young person's bed wetting were said to have been dramatic, although the cause was not known (or not divulged):

> Mrs S: It was when she was 2½ that she had this - like a nervous breakdown ... before that she was completely potty trained - both day and night - no problems - we were off nappies - nothing. And then all of a sudden, I don't know what happened, she just changed. It was like an overnight thing. She started wetting the bed, she started wetting herself, and her bowels opened as well - and she started doing the toilet up the carpet, and she'd be walking and doing the toilet at the same time - and I just couldn't cope with this. Immediately of course she got on nappies. And that's the cycle ever since.   Mother of Sarah (age 11)

Sarah was still wetting the bed on six nights per week when she entered this study. In the interim she had had problems with anorexia, she was still being seen on an occasional basis by a clinical psychologist and her weight was being regularly monitored by the paediatrician at the local hospital.

Some health care professionals researching the pathophysiology of bed wetting discount psychological disturbance as a contributory factor. However, the research of others who have compared enuretic with non-enuretic children (e.g. Jarvelin et al, 1990, 1991; Larsen and Winther, 1980; Oppel et al, 1968b) suggests that stressful life events, including divorce, parental separation, marital conflict or birth of a sibling can be precipitating factors, especially in children who have been late in acquiring primary bladder control. It has been suggested that this makes a child more susceptible to developing secondary enuresis when exposed to stressful life events (Fergusson et al, 1990). In this study some parents attributed the young person's bed wetting to the child's emotional response to a social problem between members of the family.

Day time urinary symptoms

The prevalence of day wetting for the young people in the study was high at 75 per cent but for 11 of these 15 young people the problem was said to be very occasional or occasional (Table 3.3). Seven of the young people in this study experienced a loss of day time bladder control which would be visible to others in that the leakage of urine was said to occur through to the outside of clothing. Visible loss of day time bladder control is shown to have had significant social consequences for these young people (Chapter 4).

Table 3.3

The usual frequency of bed wetting and the frequency and severity of day wetting[a]

	Age	Usual frequency of bed wetting (nights/week)	Frequency of occurrence of day wetting					Leakage of urine to outside of clothes[c]		
			Not at all	Very occasionally	Occasionally	Often	Very often	Yes	No	NA
Carol	17	7					✓	✓d		
Anthony	16	6		✓					✓	
Peter	15	6			✓				✓	
Roger	14	≤1		✓					✓	
Paul	13	3	✓							✓
Ian	13	≤1	✓							✓
Sarah	11	6		✓					✓	
Jennifer	9	4		✓					✓	
Alison	9	7					✓	✓d		
Tracy	9	5		✓					✓	
William	9	3		✓					✓	

Name									
Michelle	8	≤1	✓						✓
Simon	8	2		✓				✓	
Stephen[b]	8	7	✓			✓	✓d		
John[b]	8	3	✓						✓
Michael	8	7			✓		✓d		
Shelly	7	7			✓		✓e		
Martin	6	≤1	✓		✓				✓
Gary	5	7				✓	✓d		
Lisa	4	7					✓d		

Notes: a source of data is the urinary symptom questionnaire
  b twins
  c none of the young people wore a pad or any other from of protection to absorb any leakage of urine
  d usually
  e sometimes

Contrary to the findings of Hellstrom et al (1990), there did seem to be an association between day wetting and frequency of wet nights per week. The four young people who were reported as day wetting "very often", with the urine leaking visibly to the outside of their clothes, were also said to wet the bed seven nights per week (Table 3.3) and for three of the four young people, said to wet occasionally in the day time, the leakage was also "sometimes" or "usually" of the type which would be clearly visible to others. These seven young people had the double disadvantage of visible day as well as frequent night time problems with their bladder control which made the maintenance of secrecy impossible. Through conversations with parents and the young people themselves, it transpired that seven of the young people had recently had a day wetting episode at school, and a further four had had problems with day wetting incidents at school in the past. In contrast the five young people who had no day wetting problem only wet the bed three nights per week or less.

Summary

The families enrolled into this study have been drawn from some of the most deprived as well as the most affluent wards in the study area and include young people aged 4 to 17 years, wetting the bed from seven nights per week to less than once a week. Half these young people had experienced some form of family reorganisation. Family reordering is becoming an increasingly common phenomenon for young people in society at large.

The findings of this and other studies highlight that remarkably little is known about the natural history of the acquisition of nocturnal bladder control (Blackwell, 1992). The fundamental question remains unanswered: how many dry nights does the child need to achieve before it can be said that the physiological mechanisms required for bladder control are in place and capable of functioning reliably? The experiences of four of the sixteen families in this study, with a child originally classified as a "primary" bed wetter, suggest that there could be a "critical period" during which learning how to be dry at night can be undone, perhaps at times of stressful life events within the family. In the present study the four children who were reported by their mothers as having been reliably dry both day and night before the age of 2 to 2½ years, were aged 4, 6, 9 and 11 on entering the study. These young people were also amongst the most severely affected bed wetters.

The practical and social consequences of the young people's night and day time urinary symptoms, for themselves and for their families, are described in Chapters 4 and 5.

4 Families' experiences of bed wetting

The focus of this chapter is the family's experience a young person's bed wetting. It seeks to answer the broad research questions posed at the beginning of this study (Chapter 2). It is for the most part a descriptive account, however many of the themes and concepts described here form the building blocks of the theory developed in Chapters 5 and 6.

How do families experience the day to day practical consequences of bed wetting?

The practical, day to day consequences of bed wetting are described in this section. It is shown that the consequences of bed wetting are rarely confined to night time and can affect key times of communal family activity. Within the families the issues were different for young people of different ages. While most parents expected to help younger children, the parents of adolescents were often particularly frustrated by the young person's reluctance to take responsibility for managing those practical tasks which were deemed to be well within their capabilities.

Night time activities

Insights into night time activities relating to bed wetting were gained from three sources: the urinary symptom questionnaire; from conversations with family members, and from the diaries kept by the young people and their parents (Chapter 2).

While many of the young people may have had more than one complete micturition during the night, two thirds of them were normally unaware of having wet the bed until they woke up in the morning. In most cases their parents were also undisturbed through the night. The youngest children woke up in the night most often. However during the month of the diary keeping only four mothers were disturbed in the night because of a wet child. The majority of parents were rarely if ever disturbed.

The notable exception to this was Michael's mother. According to her diary she attended to her eight year old son's needs twice a night, on average. He had only one, partially functioning kidney and suffered from polyuria. "In the night" meant after she herself had gone to bed and before she finally got up in the morning. Her diary showed that she had changed Michael's nappy on average three times after he had gone to bed at night, ranging from twice to five times. Both Michael's parents had come to accept a situation which they believed could not be changed, being outwith Michael's control.

The diary entries of other parents reflected their feelings of frustration about the bed wetting, on some occasions, and described circumstances when disturbances relating to bed wetting could be problematic:

> MRS W: William wet when I got him up and I was annoyed because I've got myself so keyed up about my interview and I just wanted to flop into bed so I was quite abrupt with him, changed and dried him as quickly as poss. Was flustered this morning because he was wet again and I was already in a panic about the time but he had washed himself.
>
> Mother of William (age 9) Day 6 of diary

Few fathers were involved in the management of the practicalities arising from the young person's bed wetting but Paul's father was actively involved and he described similar circumstances when getting up in the night to his son was a task he could have done without:

> Mr P: The only time that's bothered me particularly has been ... in particularly stressful times workwise ... once you're awake you're not going to get back to sleep again ... that was annoying and frustrating at that stage but it didn't happen very often, so it didn't matter. But I was conscious of thinking: 'I hope to goodness it's not tonight!'
>
> Father of Paul (age 13)

These occasions tended to be memorable but for the majority of the parents, for most of the time, disturbances at night in relation to bed wetting were uncommon. It has been found that the greatest impact of bed wetting for most families, in the practical sense, is not at night but in the mornings, as family members hurriedly prepare to leave the house for school or work.

In many households with children it is quite normal for week days to start with a period of frenetic activity as children prepare to leave the house for school and many parents get ready to go to work. Many mothers said that the "morning panic" was made worse on those mornings when the young person needed extra attention because they were wet. The problem was compounded in families where a young person had wet someone else's bed as well:

> MRS L: She was wetting all the beds at night and you are up changing beds in the night and having to bath her brother before he went to school in the morning ... he was having to get up an hour early and he was getting up during his sleep. It was a shame. Mother of Lisa (age 4)

Wetting more than one bed in one night was not uncommon, being mentioned by the parents of six children. At the time of this study three families included two young people who wet the bed regularly. This compounded the work for the mothers, even when one or both of the young people was largely self-caring.

Many of the seven to nine year olds were said by their mothers to require only minimum supervision, even when they were wet. In some households a routine had been established. The younger children, however, tended to need some help, especially with their personal hygiene, and this was not always forthcoming.

Shelly was at first teased by her brother and sister, and then by the children at school because she smelt of urine:

> MRS S: There were times when she went to school you could actually smell it on her sometimes. I started washing her but when she got older and that she started doing it herself and I made sure she was clean before she went to school. They don't bother her now. Mother of Shelly (age 7)

When asked to draw a picture of how she felt in the mornings when she woke up to find herself wet Shelly drew a picture of herself in the bathroom. Shelly said that she was happy about the practicalities of managing a wet bed, such as changing the sheets and changing herself. Martin, Gary and Michelle felt much the same:

> MICHELLE: It's good - then I've not got the smell any more.
> Michelle (age 8)

One indication of the shame felt by young people, in relation to their lack of night time bladder control, is that so many had at some time tried to hide the bed wetting from their parents. In some cases the young person was frightened to admit to it:

> Mrs L: At first it was a shame because sometimes I used to get crabbit [angry], there's no point in saying I didn't, during the night she was waking me up and I said, 'for God's sake Lisa, I've not got a tumble drier, it's broken. How am I going to get these done?' I maybe got crabbit to start with ... and she would maybe be feared to tell you or she'd hide her pants - it does not bother us now.　　　　　　　　　　　　　　　Mother of Lisa (age 4)

Other children were said to have hidden wet night clothes when they had been offered a reward for achieving a certain number of dry nights.

Talking with families about the management of the consequences of bed wetting from day to day sometimes revealed a great deal about the young person's self esteem or lack of it. In contrast to the majority, Carol and Tracy gave the impression of having given up trying to help themselves, even in practical ways, expressing feelings of helplessness and hopelessness. This manifested itself as apathy when it came to managing the practical consequences of the bed wetting. The parents of both Carol and Tracy were concerned about this:

> MRS T: But she doesn't even get up, she just lies there in it.
> MOYA: What, in the urine?
> MRS T: Aye, and when she soils ... And you've got to force her to go into a bath and everything. She just doesnae - ... With Laura [the other bed wetting child in the family, age 4] when she is wet, she gets up and takes it off and jumps into Kevin's bed, whereas with Tracy, she lies in it all night ... I've got to tell her or she wouldnae do anything, you know.... it just doesn't seem to get through to her.　　　　　　　　　Mother of Tracy (age 9)

Both Carol and Tracy seemed to be unhappy about life in general, as well as being unhappy about the bed wetting.

Issues relating to the handling and laundering of the wet sheets emerged again and again as causes of irritation for some parents. The issue which caused a great deal of conflict in the families of some adolescents was who should remove the sheets. The tension surrounding this issue could carry forward through the day until the young person arrived home from school when the young person might find an angry mother and an unmade bed. These parents felt that the young person was old enough to take some responsibility for managing the practicalities and they sometimes left the bed unchanged as a matter of principle:

> MRS P: And there's been times when I thought, no, I'm just going to leave the bed, and he'll come in 4 o'clock and he brings a friend home with him - 'Is my bed made, Mum?' and I say, 'No' - and of course I rush through, give them a glass of juice and make the bed, and cover it up for him. You know you don't want to embarrass them but you know if he was making an effort it might push him a bit just to -   Mother of Peter (age 15)

In spite of her feelings of frustration Peter's mother was still concerned to protect her son from the embarrassment of discovery by others. Several mothers described their diversionary tactics as they removed the evidence of their child's bed wetting when the young person's friends called at the house.

Overall, the younger children seemed more biddable and more enthusiastic about removing the sheets than many of the older ones, who regarded it as a chore. Perhaps many of the adolescents had become apathetic about managing the wet sheets because the problem had been going on for so long, but most were still very particular about their personal hygiene and were happy to distance themselves from the problem, leaving the house and their secret behind them in the rush for school.

In summary, mornings could be a tense time for some young people when they had to face the consequences of the wet bed, and the whole family could be affected in one way or another. Mothers with younger children, who needed most help with their personal hygiene, often had most to do in the practical sense. Siblings could be affected too, if they and their bed had been made wet. It could be that some received less attention in the morning when the mother was engaged elsewhere. Most fathers were not directly involved in the practicalities but they too may have been affected by a blocked bathroom, or a harassed wife.

Dealing with one young person, who had wet one or more beds, was said to influence the atmosphere in the whole household. During the diary keeping Anthony began to experience more dry nights:

> MRS A: I do hope this lasts. Makes the atmosphere and attitude in the house normal!   Mother of Anthony (age 16) Diary entry

Many parents commented on the difference in the young person's behaviour on wet and dry mornings. On dry mornings the young person's cheerfulness and enhanced self esteem were often manifested as increased communicativeness and on some occasions led to unsolicited activity:

MRS A: Another good morning. Alison made her bed by 7 a.m. this morning, she was that pleased.   Mother of Alison (age 9)   Diary entry

MRS A: Anthony is pleased with himself. He has tieded [sic] up his bedroom for the first time without my asking saying he is 'fed up living in a mess'.   Mother of Anthony (age 16)   Diary entry

Bed time activities

From discussions with parents, bed times did not emerge as particularly problematic times in most families, except during family holidays when special preparations were deemed to be necessary to protect someone else's bed. It appeared that at home routines had been established which the young person and their parents were confident would minimise the consequences of bed wetting, for the most part, and at home no one outwith the family was involved.

In most families the young person's bed was protected with a plastic sheet placed between the mattress and the bottom sheet. This caused many practical problems. Many young people found that they were too hot at night. Lisa's mother described how everyone in the household had suffered from this as Lisa was one of those children who sometimes wet several beds in one night:

Mrs L: We all had covers on our beds ... it attracts the heat and everybody's sweating and you cannot sleep all night. So we ended up taking them off our bed, and told her she wasn't to come in to our bed, because we have just got a new bed and I thought 'I cannot keep up with this'.   Mother of Lisa (age 4)

Many mothers found the plastic sheets difficult to clean and dry and were concerned that there was always a residual odour. Two mothers described how the plastic sheets had disintegrated when put in the washing machine. Other mothers had tried scrubbing the plastic sheeting - the result was holes.

In the light of all the practical problems associated with the use of plastic sheeting it is not surprising that some mothers had resorted to putting the young person back into nappies. This practice sometimes started at a holiday time, in the attempt to try to prevent the embarrassment of the young person wetting someone else's bed:

MRS L: At first it was terrible to try and get her to wear nappies. Oh it was really terrible. As you were putting them on her she was pulling them off. I said, 'Lisa, you have to' - it was on holiday last year we started

66

wearing them. I said, 'You're in someone else's bed' sort of thing. The first couple of nights she greeted [cried], but after that she sort of - 'Oh well, if I've got to wear them, I've got to wear them'. And she has worn them ever since.   Mother of Lisa (age 4)

The health visitor had given Sarah (age 11) nappies to take on a school holiday to save her the embarrassment of discovery, but Sarah's mother had attempted to continue with the practice at home afterwards. Sarah did not express much emotion when the topic came up during conversation but she had obviously been unhappy about the practice and her mother discovered that she had discontinued with their use. In conversation about the body worn alarm, which Sarah was refusing to use because she said it was "babyish", the nappies were alluded to again:

MRS S: She says that ['it's babyish'] about the nappies as well and I told her she either stops or she uses them.   Mother of Sarah (age 11)

Martin's mother had taken an equally uncompromising position:

MRS M: But I know when my mother-in-law found out, she found out last year and she was horrified. She says, 'get nappies off him and just bring the wet sheets round every day and I'll wash them'. I mean, I get on fine with her, but it wasn't me she said it to, but my husband, and I says, 'If she wants wet sheets every day she can have them because I'm not doing it'. Even now, if he wasn't dry now, he'd be back in them because there's no way, I'm not washing every day! It's bad enough when there is an accident.
                                   Mother of Martin (age 6)

Three other mothers had tried to shame their sons into being dry by putting them into a nappy on just one occasion. Gary's mother had not persisted with this approach because of the consequences:

MRS G: ...I thought he was gonnae take a fit, and it was disturbin' tae see him ... I was nearly greetin' [crying] fur him. ... You'd think I had killed him. And he was actually heartbroken, and he was embarrassed, and he was - his heid was ready to blow off his shoolders. He was hysterical ... So I just thought, well, that's no' the answer.
                                    Mother of Gary (age 5)

Whether through trial and error or intuition the majority of mothers recognised that the use of nappies in children over the age of three or four was humiliating for the child. Children as young as four years old, such as Lisa and Gary, had exhibited signs of acute distress on being put back into nappies after a period of time without them. For those children who were made to wear nappies over a prolonged period, their feelings of embarrassment and shame at bed times can only be imagined, as they were reminded of their inability to do what they believed most three year olds could do - namely keep their bed and themselves dry through the night.

In this study it has been difficult to gauge whether the anticipation of the possibility of wetting the bed affected the feelings and behaviour of the young people at bed time, when nappies were not in use. However some light was shed on the question when Simon became dry after completing the urinary symptom questionnaire. His mother had no doubt about the effect that being reliably dry for two weeks had had on Simon's demeanour at bed time:

> MRS S: I think he's a changed child in a couple of weeks, quite honestly. If I say to him, 'It's time to go to bed', he goes to bed. We don't have this sort of messing around and getting cross and stomping around. He still does that when he's tired, he's been up late, but he's easier. You're an easier boy (to Simon). You're a happier boy. He comes down in the morning, big smile on his face, he's dry.   Mother of Simon (age 8)

What part do the different family members play in the management of the young person's bed wetting?

The mother as orchestrator

In 17 of the 19 families the mother clearly played the major part in helping the young person with the management of the day to day practicalities arising from the bed wetting, as well as supervising any treatments tried. They managed situations involving others outwith the household such as wider family, friends and health care professionals. Most mothers acted as the "orchestrator" of events, co-ordinating the activities of people within and outwith the household.

It so happened that most mothers in the first families to be enrolled were actively involved in seeking solutions to the young person's bed wetting at the time of the study. Many had developed a conscious strategy for handling the situation which reflected their beliefs about the cause of the bed wetting and the young person's control over it. However, it transpired that even within the more proactive families there were long periods when no treatment was actively being sought. At these times the parents tended to fall back on established evening and night time routines. These were, for the most part, supervised by the mother. In three families recruited late into this study there was much less evidence of an overall strategy or of consciously planned action to seek to resolve the bed wetting. The parents in these families merely seemed to be responding to events from day to day. However, even in these families, the mother was still responsible for helping the young person with the practicalities arising from the bed wetting from day to day.

The socialisation of women into the role of "mother" has been described, for instance, by Graham (1986, 1993); Oakley (1979); Urwin (1985) and Wetherell (1995). In every society there are certain implicit and explicit expectations of a mother's behaviour. In her book *The Ideology of Motherhood* Wearing (1984, p.49) describes the "good" mother:

> A good mother is one who is always available to her children; she gives time and attention to them, listens to their problems and questions and guides them where necessary. She cares for them physically ... She is calm and patient, does not scream or yell or continually smack her children. The cardinal sin of motherhood with its associated guilt is to lose one's temper with a child. Self-control should be exercised at all times. Even in extenuating circumstances ... when the mother has no emotional or physical support in her task, she must at all times be in complete control of her own emotions.

Wearing acknowledges that an unrealistically high standard is set by such an ideal. It suggests that the mother should always put the young person's interests above her own.

Wetherell (1995) suggests that the mother is seen by society as the parent who is primarily responsible for a child's welfare and is expected to provide consistently high quality parenting, regardless of the degree of social and relational stress she is experiencing. Wetherell suggests that failure to live up to the ideal can result in a mother feeling guilty and a failure. Many of the mothers in this study expressed feelings of guilt after they had punished their child for wetting the bed and two mothers expressed the view that health care professionals blamed them for the young person's bed wetting.

Overall the mother's role in the management of the young person's bed wetting was not seen to be an easy one. The consequences of bed wetting could make physical and emotional demands on mothers at key times of communal family activity, such as the morning rush for school. There were also social and emotional consequences of the bed wetting for family relationships more generally, when a mother could find herself in the role of arbitrator, as is described later in this chapter.

The father's role

From talking with parents and the young people in this study five patterns of paternal involvement emerged:

- the father was rarely, if ever, involved

- the father was occasionally involved in a few specific ways

- the father had become increasingly involved in the search for a solution to the bed wetting but the mother was largely responsible for managing the practicalities from day to day

- the mother and father shared both the overall responsibility and the day to day care on an equitable basis, according to their availability

- the father had abdicated responsibility for care and "didn't want to know", leaving the mother to manage alone.

In four of these five patterns the mother was regarded by both parents as being in overall control.

Four young people had two father figures in their lives, their natural father, with whom they stayed on occasion, and a step-father or the mother's male partner with whom they stayed for the majority of time. This gave rise to a sixth pattern of occasional paternal involvement. Examples of each pattern of paternal involvement and the context in which each arose are now described.

Ten of the twelve fathers interviewed for this study said that they were rarely or only occasionally involved in caring for their bed wetting child in the practical sense:

> MR. W:...quite often I wake up, maybe before Lorna certainly, but I usually just wake up Lorna. She does that ... I don't really do anything to do with that ... I just book the holidays, so to speak (laughs). [William's father was a travel agent]   Stepfather of William   (age 9)

Shelly's father was a garage mechanic:

> MOYA: Do you get involved at all?
> MR S: No. She does (he laughs, looking at his wife). I'm out there [in his garage] near enough 24 hours a day.
>   Father of Shelly (age 7)

Three mothers commented that their partners were not available for child care of any kind because they worked long hours. In two cases, where the parents were divorced, the mother said that the natural father had taken no part in the care.

Four mothers said that the father was, or had in the past, been occasionally involved in specific ways, most usually in lifting the child at the parents' own bed time. The father's involvement in this way occurred in some families once the young person was too heavy for the mother to lift. Occasionally the father's help was invoked if the mother felt that a firmer hand was needed.

The data suggest that as the young person grows older, some fathers become more involved in seeking solutions to the problem at their wives' request. The mothers in these families were still said to be responsible for the day to day practicalities:

> MR P: Well, Louise [his wife] basically is the one that's dealing with Peter most of the time. When there's been - when I've come in at night and we've tried to waken him up - things like that - that's really my involvement in it. My involvement's not been a great deal.   Father of Peter   (age 15)

Fathers in this category were, however, said to be willing to help if asked.

Only two fathers in this study were said to have consistently shared responsibility for managing the everyday consequences of the young person's bed wetting. Paul's mother had suffered from post-natal depression after both her sons were born and Paul's father had taken a great deal of responsibility for caring for his sons, in practical ways, since they were babies. In the only other case where a father had accepted many of the day to day responsibilities associated with the bed wetting, the father had been unemployed for three years. His wife worked part time and he had taken on many of the domestic tasks. This family was particularly accepting of the situation. Both parents shared the same philosophy, as well as the care. When asked what advice they would give to other parents, they said:

> MR I: There's no point in taking it out on the wean [child].
> MRS I: It's not their problem, it's not their fault.
> MR I: It's going to stop.
> MRS I: It's just waiting.   Parents of Ian (age 13)

The sense of partnership was reflected in these parents' replies to many questions. Ian's mother had wet the bed herself until she was 11 years old.

Three fathers were not as involved with the young person's care or as supportive of their wives as were the fathers of Ian, Paul, Anthony and Peter, nor indeed, did it seem that they wished to be. These fathers were said by the mothers to be very angry about the bed wetting, to want it to stop, but to want nothing to do with helping it to stop. They didn't want to know. In two cases the father was said to have little positive involvement with the child in other ways:

> MRS G: Alan's never been a part of their life as in taking them away tae a park, or takin' them a walk, or takin' them tae visit his family - the bairns' life revolve roond me, 24 hoors a day.　　　　　Mother of Gary　(age 5)

Another father was said to have resented the attention that the young person had received from his wife:

> MRS C: My ex-husband didn't like the idea of me getting up out of my bed, lifting her up to the toilet and putting her back. He didn't like that at all. He said she was nothing but a lazy - he called her lazy ... I said leave her and she'll come out of it. He wanted me for himself.
> 　　　　　　　　　　　　　　　　　　　　Mother of Carol (age 17)

Carol's father wet the bed himself:

> MRS C: It was worse when he had a drink in him ... It was two or three times a week sometimes, and I says - and he kept shouting at me, at Carol, lifting Carol to the toilet.　　　　　　　　Mother of Carol (age 17)

After separating from his wife and leaving the family home, this father sexually abused his daughter for three years, from the age of 11 to 14 on her weekend visits to him and he was imprisoned for it.

In each of these three families the relationship between the parents was said by the mother to be or to have been poor and the tensions in the house were said to be or to have been high. In each case the young person was thought by the father to have more control over the bed wetting than he or she was choosing to exercise and all these children had been punished for it over a prolonged period.

The involvement of fathers no longer living within the household In those cases where the mother had re-married or had a new partner she was quite clearly the orchestrator of events, co-ordinating the activities of others within and outwith the household. Two mothers, who were themselves against the use of punishment for bed wetting, felt that the natural fathers' attitude was unhelpful when the children stayed with them at weekends:

MRS S: ... I don't think his dad and his gran were particularly clued into what the problem was and he was put back into a nappy one time, and then I think there was a bit of a stigma if there was a wet bed ... Messages like, 'Well I'm not going to wash the sheets every night' sort of thing, didn't help things. In fact it was a disaster.   Mother of Simon (age 8)

MRS J: I was taking them back, like, [after a weekend visit to the natural father] and he used to crack up with them because they'd wet the bed, and I said, 'You used to do it'. He says, 'Aye, I ken, but I still -'. He was angry at them because they wet the bed.

Mother of John and Stephen (twins, age 8)

It is worthy of note in the second example, that the unsympathetic father was known to have been a bed wetter himself. It was not known whether Simon's father had wet the bed. In this study there is evidence to suggest that most mothers who were bed wetters themselves were particularly accepting of their child's predicament, whereas some fathers who had been bed wetters were clearly not.

The father's role in child care more generally The findings of this study are congruent with the findings of more general research into child care, which shows that the mother normally has most responsibility for child care on a day to day basis (Demo and Acock, 1993; Gelles, 1995; Graham, 1993; Muncie et al, 1995).

During the last 30 years men's participation in the paid labour force has significantly declined while the proportion of married women in the work force has risen sharply, albeit mostly in part time employment (Hood, 1993). The most striking change has been the increase in employed mothers, especially the mothers of babies and pre-school children (Hoffman, 1989; Menaghan and Parcel, 1990). During this time there has been an increasing interest in the father's role in child care (e.g. Biller, 1993; Cohen, 1993; Daly, 1993; Stier and Tienda, 1993). However, there is some disagreement among researchers about the extent to which men's involvement in household work and child care has increased in the last three decades during the time when women's working lives have changed dramatically.

Some studies have found a slight increase in the proportion of family work undertaken by husbands whose wives are employed (Pleck, 1985). Other researchers claim that there has been little increase in men's house work and child care activities (Coverman and Sheley (1986). Goldscheider and Waite (1991) found that even in homes where both husband and wife worked, the wife undertook more of the household work and child care activities.

Rexroat and Sheehan (1987) found that women worked longer hours than men at every stage in the family life cycle but especially when the family included children under three years old. "Work" included both paid employment and looking after the home and children. This unequal division of labour was confirmed by Hochschild and Machung (1989) who calculated that many wives were working an extra "shift", amounting to nearly an extra month of work per year.

Both parents worked full time in only one of the 19 families in the present study. In this family the wife was clearly responsible for all matters relating to child care, although her working day was at least as long as her husband's. In the present study all but two of the mothers regarded themselves, and were regarded by their husbands, as the principal carer in the practical sense. Management of bed wetting did not seem to be regarded as a special case but as a natural extension of the mother's more general child care role.

It has been found that mothers spend more time than fathers with their children in middle childhood and adolescence (Russell and Russell, 1987), as well as in early childhood. Stafford and Bayer (1993) suggest that even once their children are largely self-caring mothers talk with their children more and over a greater range of topics than is the case for most fathers. They suggest that fathers' conversations are characterised by a control function, and are concerned with issues of discipline and setting boundaries, while mother-adolescent interactions are more likely to involve personal and social issues. In the present study while many parents remarked that they talked with their children about their bed wetting from time to time, the researcher wondered whether some young people felt able to talk about their bed wetting with anyone at all within the family.

A review of the recent literature suggests that within and across cultures the expectations of fathers are more varied than the expectations of mothers. "Good" fathers have been variously defined as: patriarchs, disciplinarians, moral educators, educators about the ways of the world, their children's best friend and substitute mothers (Harris and Morgan, 1991; Biller, 1993; Cohen, 1993; Daly, 1993; Deutsch et al, 1993; Haas, 1993; Holland, 1994; Hood, 1993; Ishii-Kuntz, 1993; Stier and Tienda, 1993). Haas (1993) clearly describes the influence of social policy on the father's role in Sweden. Culturally defined expectations of fathers to take equal responsibility with their wives for many aspects of child care in Sweden contrasts sharply with the authoritarian ideal in Japan where child care is seen almost exclusively as the mother's role (Ishii-Kuntz, 1993). Expectations of fathers in Britain seem to lie somewhere in between.

All the young people in this study were living in families with at least one brother or sister. As members of a family with a young person who wet the bed siblings were, at the least, observers of events and were often affected themselves, directly or indirectly. The practical consequences were greatest for the seven children who shared a bedroom with a bed wetter. Some siblings may have received less attention in the morning rush for school as the parents were engaged elsewhere. Some were disturbed in the night when the young person was receiving treatment with a body worn alarm. Many were undoubtedly affected by the practical arrangements relating to family holidays, and the restrictions imposed on choice and type of holiday. However few were involved with the management of the practicalities arising from the bed wetting from day to day in anything more than a passing way.

None of the young people in this study shared a bed with a sibling, but two younger sisters of one of them did and one of them was a bed wetter. Anne (age 7) who did wet the bed described her sister's obvious displeasure at her bed wetting:

> MOYA: ... What does Linda say when she wakes up and finds a wet patch? ...
> ANNE: She fights with me.

William's mother could still clearly remember what it was like to share a bed with a bed wetter:

> MRS W: I was actually sharing a bed with her, because she was younger and we were, you know, all in the same room, and she used to wet me ... I can remember I used to get up and I'd say, 'Oh, not again!', and she used to sit there and say, 'I'm really, really sorry. I had a dream I was going to the toilet, and I was still in my bed!'   Mother of William (age 9)

It could be that in some parts of Britain it is more common for children to share a bed than was the case in the present study (Karandikar, 1992). Such bed wetters face the potential disapproval of their siblings on every occasion when the bed is wet, which could well reinforce their feelings of embarrassment and shame.

It is impossible, however, for a young person to avoid the censure of others, even when they only share a room. Michelle's mother could remember what it was like to share a room with a bed wetter until her sister was 14 years old:

MRS M: It was hard, we shared a room, you could smell the bed in the morning, and it was horrible ... In the mornings you could see her making the bed and I would go and say 'Is your bed dry?' 'Oh aye', but she was hiding it, she was getting embarrassed about it.'

Mother of Michelle (age 8)

The maternal grandfathers of William and of the twins, John and Stephen, were said to have abdicated all responsibility for the management of the bed wetting in the way that some fathers in this study were said to have abdicated responsibility. The consequences for William's mother, her bed wetting sister and their mother were particularly far reaching and lasted for nearly six years. This is a case where a sibling had a special part to play in the day to day practicalities:

MRS W: She got to about 8 or 9, and my father said, 'look, you know, this is it, she's going to stop and you'd better make her stop' - and my mother was left to you know sort of arrange it herself, and what she actually did was, she got a buzzer for her, but it used to be a big pack machine ... I don't know how it worked because my mother never had it on, because when the buzzer went off it was an almighty zzzzzzzzzzz - like a siren - she couldn't use it because my father would have heard it and then he would have known that she hadn't still stopped wetting the bed. My mother covered it up - it was a big secret ... my mother couldn't even wash the sheets or anything when my dad was in because then he would have known. I couldn't go through and knock my mother's door in the middle of the night because then he would have known. I used to have to get up with her, change her, change the bed, put the two of us back into bed ... and my mother used to put you know sheets and everything in the bottom of the cupboard so I could just get up without my dad knowing. So of course my dad lived in blissful ignorance from about the time she was 8, and she never stopped till she was 14, and it was hidden ...

Mother of William (age 9)

This was the only example to be uncovered in this study of secrecy being maintained within a subsystem of the family. William's mother clearly described the anxiety and tension that this situation created for her mother, her sister and herself. It is extraordinary that the women in the house managed to keep the secret for so long. Paternal intolerance to bed wetting was discovered in the present study. The above historical example may not merely be a reflection of a by-gone era.

What are the social consequences of bed wetting from the young person's perspective?

The social consequences of bed wetting are reviewed in this section from the young person's perspective, with special reference to the consequences for the young person's relationships with siblings and friends. It was discovered that many young people had to face the censure of their siblings from day to day, especially if they shared a bedroom. Most young people were afraid of the consequences of people outwith the household discovering that they wet the bed. Some young people denied that even their closest friends knew about the bed wetting, which was a closely guarded secret. Many young people were anxious about staying away from home for this reason.

Relationships with siblings

All the young people in this study were living in families with at least one brother or sister. Most of the young people were very hesitant in their response to any questions about how their siblings felt about the bed wetting. Five said that their younger brothers and sisters did not know about it.

Peter said that his younger half brother (aged 2½), who was already dry at night, was "too young" to know about it, a fact denied by his parents in a later conversation:

> MRS P: You were asking Peter the other night, 'What do the rest of the family feel about it?' And he said, 'Och, Stuart's too young' - and I thought I should have said to you then, Stuart's even said to him - 'Oh, is Peter's bed wet?' because he's even paying attention to it now ... if I go through and if I change it the odd time, and I strip it or whatever- 'Peter's wet his bed - you're not supposed to wet your bed, are you' - I say - 'No'.
>
> Mother of Peter (age 15)

In two cases older siblings were said to be happy because they were able to use the bed wetting as an opportunity to "score points":

> MOYA: How does your oldest brother feel about it?
> ROGER: Happy, so he can slag me.   Roger (age 14)

Many of the young people felt vulnerable to being put down by older siblings because of the bed wetting. The two children who felt that their younger brothers and sisters were very unhappy about the bed wetting shared the same bedroom:

MARTIN: ... he doesn't like me wetting the bed.
MOYA: Does he not? What does he say to you?
MARTIN: 'Go away, Martin'.   Martin   (age 6)

Shelly (age 7) believed that her brother and sister were unhappy about the bed
wetting too and they called her names. The negative attitude of many siblings
to the young person's bed wetting may well reinforce the young person's
feelings of embarrassment and shame. It is a situation from which there is no
easy escape, especially in those families whose sleeping accommodation is
limited and sharing a bedroom is unavoidable.

The fear of discovery and rejection by others

Maintaining secrecy was high on the agenda for most of the young people in
this study. This became apparent even in response to a question about the
young person's feelings about taking part in this study:

IAN: I'm not bothered what folk kens as long as my pals don't find out.
                                                                   Ian (age 13)

When asked what their special friends felt about the bed wetting five of the
young people said that none of their friends knew, three evaded the question
and five gave a non-committal reply. Two young people, who admitted that
they had a special friend who knew about it, spontaneously added that they
were sure that this friend would keep the knowledge a secret:

MOYA: Do any of your friends know about it? (he shakes his head) ...
How do you think they would feel if they did know?
JOHN: Well there's one of my pals that knows, that's my really really best
friend and he's not opened his mouth ... He doesn't say anything. He just ...
MOYA: Do you ever talk about it?
JOHN: I talked about it - I says to him once, 'How would you feel if you
wet the bed?' and he said he would feel the same as what I feel.
                                                                   John (age 8)

MOYA: Do any of your friends know about it?
MICHELLE: One friend ... Cos, I know I can trust her. And she says,
'Right, I'll tell not one person'. She always tells me the truth ... she says
'You have to stop it, everybody will find out sooner or later'.
                                                              Michelle (age 8)

Peter and Michael found it hard to talk to any friends about it, even, in one case, when the friend was also a bed wetter:

> PETER: Before I moved here I had a best friend - he done exactly the same - he knew, we knew each other.
> MOYA: Yes. So you talked about it?
> PETER: No! We never talked about it! - we just knew we did.
> Peter (age 15)

> MICHAEL: ... friends normally tell everybody about things - but I don't tell my friend about it.
> Michael (age 8)

Although there was a known cause for the bed wetting, Michael, a very sociable child, was still reluctant to talk about it with his closest friends. As with the other young people he felt ashamed about a problem over which he believed he had no control.

In the light of the response of their siblings, in some cases, and the humiliation experienced when bladder control was lost in public in the day time, the reason for the desire to maintain secrecy was not hard to imagine:

> MRS J: I had to go up to the school. He was saying that the teacher wasn't letting him out to the toilet. But when Stephen needs, he needs. He's just got to go. I had said to her at the beginning of the year, that he needed to go. And he was coming in and he was wet. And it got to the stage that he was coming home greeting [crying]. He was coming home, breaking his heart and he was wanting long tops to hide it because they were all making fun of him, but she wasn't letting him out - 'Do your work first', and he was slow anyway, ken.
> Mother of Stephen   (age 8)

Roger commented with some feeling on the injustice of the social consequences of bed wetting for an older person:

> ROGER: And I saw a film about this old guy who pee'd the bed at night, and his family wouldn't have him, and his wife and all that died, and he had kids. And they wouldn't let him stay with them ... and I was shouting at the film, 'It's not right, it's not right!'
> Roger (age 14)

Great care was taken in this study not to raise the possible long-term consequences of bed wetting with these young people and their parents. By the time of this study, Roger was fortunately nearly dry and the problem was perceived by him and his family as nearly over. It is not known whether any of the other young people had gained any insights into the possible long-term consequences of bed wetting, such as social isolation and homelessness. Sarah's mother had asked the age range of the young people taking part in this study. In response to the reply "5 to 20 years old" she said that if Sarah was still wetting the bed when she was 20, she would be "out of the house". There is no way of knowing how seriously this comment was made, or what Sarah's mother would do if that time came.

Problems relating to staying away from home and having friends to stay

When asked what the best thing would be about being reliably dry five young people gave a social benefit. They said that they looked forward to being able to have friends to stay or to being able to stay away from home without fear of discovery. Even when the bed wetting seemed to be well controlled, the fear of loss of control was still at the back of some young people's minds:

> IAN: You ken you'll no' wet the bed with that Desmospray, but you're just worried a wee bit in case you do - it doesn't work, or something.
>
> Ian (age 13)

Jennifer was really looking forward to staying away from home when she was dry but as things were she was reluctant to take the risk:

> JENNIFER: I can't really stay at my friend's house ... she always asks me to stay at her house, and I say 'No'. And she asks me why, and I say 'I just don't like staying at other people's houses'. Jennifer (age 9)

The literature on the psychosocial consequences of bed wetting for young people emphasises their negative feelings about staying away from home (Chapter 1) but in this study seven young people said that they enjoyed their trips away. Two of the seven were amongst the most frequent bed wetters. It may be that the seven young people who enjoyed staying away from home were doing so in an uncritical environment, where those around them had learned to cope unobtrusively with the bed wetting or it could be that for these young people the social pleasures of staying away from home outweighed any fear of discovery. It was not merely age related. Although most of the young people who were happy about staying away from home were aged nine or younger, other children of the same age were unhappy about doing so. It has not proved possible to explain fully the polarity of feelings about staying away from home expressed by the young people in this study, but it did appear that those who were reluctant to stay away, while a dry bed could not be assured, were those who feared or had come most to fear the consequences of discovery. This could be as much related to their personality as to the positive or negative nature of any actual experiences of staying away from home that they had had. It is also possible that some young people had learned to fear possible humiliation when staying away from home from their parents' reluctance to let them go.

What are the social consequences of bed wetting for the family as a social system?

This section draws together many of the themes highlighted so far in this chapter by considering the consequences of bed wetting for relationships within the family and the outside influences impinging on the family as a social unit.

The place of bed wetting on the family's agenda and its effects on relationships within the family

As the "architects" of the family (Yerby et al, 1995 p.16), parents are generally in overall control of the family as a social unit and determine, to a considerable extent, the priority assigned to items on the family's agenda for action. The priority assigned to a young person's bed wetting by the parents may not reflect its priority in the eyes of the young person who may be, or feel, unable to articulate the depth of his or her concern about it.

The distinction therefore needs to be made between bed wetting as an issue of collective family concern, which is largely identified as such by the parents, and bed wetting as an ongoing cause of concern for most young people, who may remain silent, feeling helpless to do anything about it themselves and reluctant to discuss it within the family because of their feelings of embarrassment and shame (Chapter 5).

At the time of the study, the parents of Ian, Shelly and Simon said that they did not regard the young person's bed wetting as an issue in the family. Parents in most of the remaining families said that they were frustrated by the bed wetting and wanted it to stop but said that they had accepted, or had come to accept it, as a fact of life:

MRS W: The way I look at it is, it's a problem that will solve itself eventually, we don't know how long it will take, but eventually he will come out of it. So there's no point in getting upset.

Mother of William (age 9)

81

These parents believed that one day the bed wetting would stop, even if they could not be sure when this would happen. However, one or both parents in each of these families recounted one or more times in the family's history when they had been less philosophical about the bed wetting, which had then been placed much higher on the family's list of priorities for action:

> MRS M: I had went to the doctor and I'd went to the health visitor and I feel I've asked that many people that I can about the situation. It was like - it had become an obsession. It really was a problem. It wasn't just once a night, but if anyone had come in and he was sitting with a nappy on - wandering about in his nappy ... I thought that there would be no end to this! That's how down I was because I thought, 'This is never going to end!' It was quite a big thing in our lives.   Mother of Martin (age 6)

The mothers of Alison and Jennifer had felt equally desperate and helpless until they realised that the young person had no control over the situation and they had also come to believe that the problem would resolve itself in time. Before coming to this realisation, the mothers of Martin, Alison and Jennifer had punished their children for wetting the bed and there was said to have been a great deal of tension in these households on "wet" mornings.

Some parents said that the bed wetting had been a particular problem for them, and for relationships within the family in the past, at a time or times when other stressful events were occurring. At these times the young person's bed wetting could become a focus for angry exchanges between the parents:

> MRS L: At first it caused a lot of rows because he thought - he was worse than me - 'She's lazy', she's this and that, 'She's not getting any more juice'. But now it's just another part of life. It's not a great big deal any more.
> Mother of Lisa (age 4)

Five of the mothers in this study said that they had had a long-standing health problem which at times pushed the bed wetting up their agenda, because of their reduced ability to cope with it.

A cause of tension within the household which was directly attributable to the young person's bed wetting was the cost of the extra laundry and the practical problems of drying bedding in winter time in Scotland. This was a particular cause of concern for families when they were short of money. The situation was particularly acute for Michael's parents because of his chronic renal problems, which included both day and night time wetting.

The way in which one young person's bed wetting could affect the relationship between siblings is described earlier in this chapter. In one family sibling rivalry also seemed to have affected the relationship between each young person and the mother. The parents were well aware of the situation:

> MRS A: (aside to Susan) Why do you pick on him for it? You'll make money out of it.
> SUSAN: How do I? Make money? (sounds very affronted)
> MRS A: Not money - you make - what's the word I was thinking of? When you have brother and sisterly love, when you try to score points against your brother -
> SUSAN: Oh well, he scores points off me as much as I score points off him!
> Mother and sister of Anthony (age 16)

Anthony had been wetting the bed six nights per week on average at the start of the study, according to the urinary symptom questionnaire, but this fell to an average of two nights per week for the month of the diary keeping. His mother said that during this month she had given her son extra attention and affection but that this had had an unfortunate and unforeseen side effect:

> MRS A: Anthony felt good about it himself and dry again. Still getting on well with Anthony but Susan seems to feel left out as she and I have always had a good relationship. You can never win, can you?
> Mother of Anthony (age 16) Diary entry

It transpired that Susan had been annoyed by the extra attention that Anthony had received during the diary keeping and had, at one point, refused to say more than the occasional word to her mother. Anthony's mother felt that she was being forced to choose between her children. She valued her close relationship with her daughter. After the diary keeping was completed, Anthony reverted to wetting the bed nearly every night of the week.

The "meaning" that Susan attached to the extra attention that Anthony received from their mother during the diary keeping altered Susan's behaviour towards her mother and ultimately the behaviour of this mother towards her son. This is a good example of Yerby et al's (1995) suggestion that family members are connected to one another by "rubber bands". Movement between two members of the family can cause re-alignment of all family members but if this movement is opposed, as it was by Susan, relationships can revert to the status quo.

In the light of the data presented throughout this chapter it is suggested that any understanding of the nature of a family's experience of bed wetting and their responses to it need to be seen in the context of relationships within the family more generally. This has important implications for practice, especially where pre-existing family dynamics could hinder the creation of a supportive environment for the young person to learn, or relearn the skill of becoming dry at night (Chapter 6).

The data support the findings of Haque et al (1981) and Devlin and O'Cathain (1990) that not all families are equally concerned about the young person's bed wetting (Chapter 1). The negative and pervasive consequences of bed wetting for some families in this study are at one extreme but important end of a continuum of experience. At the other end of the continuum there are some families who regard themselves as unaffected or only minimally affected by the bed wetting. Most families seem to be at a point on the continuum somewhere in between these two extremes.

Parents' unease about letting the young person stay away from home

Many parents in this study said that they had felt uneasy about allowing the young person the freedom of staying away from home. Many expressed the concern that the young person would be hurt by the reaction of others to the bed wetting. Some parents also commented on the embarrassment to themselves arising from the need to forewarn others of the possibility of a bed wetting episode. The embarrassment was said to arise because of other people's expectations:

MRS W: People expect, if he's 9, that he should have been out of that years ago. Whereas I mean I know from my sister that my sister went on till she was about 14, so it just doesn't work that way.
Mother of William (age 9)

Anthony's parents had been hesitant about letting their son go on a school trip abroad, because of the bed wetting and their worst fears came true:

MRS A: At 7 o'clock one morning we had a phone call from Germany to say that Anthony had wet the bed!
MR A: Well I think it was a bit more explicit than that! ...
SUSAN: Mummy was threatening to have him flown back and things.
MRS A: I was hysterical. I have friends who have relatives out there -
MR A: What can you do at 7 ... in the morning, from 700 miles away?
MRS A: Exactly. They were prepared to go and to pick him up and bring him back... Fancy phoning up at 7 o'clock - about a situation I already knew, that I was on tenterhooks about anyway.
Mother, father and sister of Anthony (age 16)

Anthony was very publicly humiliated in front of his peers. In fact Anthony's whole family was humiliated by this experience and the parents had felt helpless to intervene because he was so far from home. This and similar stories illustrate how much young people and their families are at the mercy of the attitude of others.

The effect of such incidents on a young person's self-esteem may be considerable. Certainly, such incidents were long remembered by the whole family. There may be much justification for parents' reluctance to allow a young person, who wets the bed, to stay away from home without them.

Families' experiences of the attitudes of wider family

Many young people's first experience of staying away from home without their parents involves going to stay with relatives who live nearby. This might seem a safer option than entrusting a young person to adults who are not so well known to the family, but for some young people this was not an available option. Three mothers said that their relatives were not happy about having the young person to stay until the bed wetting had stopped:

> MRS L: Nobody will let her stay, she doesn't stay at her auntie's because she wets the bed, not that I think she would, because she would be embarrassed by somebody else putting a nappy on. Mother of Lisa (age 4)

Lisa had in fact stayed with her aunt on one occasion when her mother was in hospital. She had wet the bed and had been afraid to tell anyone.

When analysing the attitudes of grandparents to the young person's bed wetting an inter-generational tendency was observed. In two cases where the grandparents were intolerant of the bed wetting the parents (their children) held a similarly intolerant view:

> MRS T: My mum'll not let her stay especially - she says she's a bed wetter. She says when - 'Once you stop that you can come and stay here'.
> Mother of Tracy (age 9)

In contrast, in several other cases the parents and grandparents appeared to be equally tolerant of the situation. In Shelly's family there seemed to be a general acceptance of the bed wetting:

> MOYA: And what's the family attitude to it?
> MRS S: Not really blaming her, but just, they've just accepted it as well.
> Mother of Shelly (age 9)

Although she was unhappy about the bed wetting Shelly was happy about staying away from home.

The few uncles whose views were commented upon by the parents seemed to have been less sympathetic with the young person than the aunts were, in a way which is reminiscent of the more negative feelings expressed by some fathers, especially those fathers who had wet the bed themselves. Problems could arise when a male relative came to stay. William's mother strongly disapproved of her brother's attitude:

> MRS W: Their [men's] attitude is, he should have stopped wetting the bed. And my brother's really bad for that, cos he comes home from college at the weekends ... and he says 'You know you should be out of that by now and you're going to be a man soon, we can't have you wetting the bed' ... Gives him - you know - five minutes, you know - macho talk, and floats out and sees him in a month's time you know ... Oh, I've told him, I said 'I don't want you talking to him like that', you know, because I think, well, he probably won't take any notice, but then again he might.
>
> Mother of William (age 9)

This is a clear example of maternal protectiveness. There were other examples of a mother protecting a bed wetting child from his or her adult male relatives, including the young person's father.

While most parents believed that the young person was unaware of the negative attitudes of relatives to the bed wetting it would be surprising if at least some of these young people had not become aware of these attitudes, whether through overhearing conversations, through non-verbal cues such as a disapproving face, or indirectly when they were not invited to stay.

Problems associated with staying away from home as a family

It is perhaps not surprising, in the light of the foregoing description of some young people's experiences of staying away from home, that many of the families said that they chose self-catering holidays when they went away together as a family, to avoid the embarrassment of having to explain the situation to other people. Several parents commented that such a holiday required some extra preparations such as packing extra sheets and an extra duvet or a sleeping bag. The inconvenience of extra laundry when away from home and home facilities was also mentioned.

So concerned were some young people and their parents about the possibility of a wet bed that they slept very poorly indeed:

MRS J: ... basically I think she's frightened to sleep.

JENNIFER: I sort of sleep with one eye open!

MRS J: Basically I think, if we go anywhere like a hotel or that, she is frightened to sleep. I'm like that as well and I feel you just don't enjoy it.

Jennifer (age 9) and her mother

Jennifer's mother commented that she often fell asleep in the afternoons when on holiday. It is not surprising, perhaps, that many families said that they felt more tired after the holiday than before it. The inability to relax at night time was an obvious contributory factor.

When families did stay in hotels or bed and breakfast accommodation a factor which emerged as a major determinant of the nature of the experience was the attitude of the people with whom the family stayed:

MRS M: We used to go camping - we had a trailer tent - this year we went to a hotel - but the people knew the situation and they were fabulous - they were really good. We always take our own bedding and an extra duvet and whatnot, but - the man was absolutely wonderful with him. Michael doesn't eat when he's not feeling well, ... and poor Dave was making things for his dinner, you know, special things whereas it was, you know, the [set] evening meal, Dave said, 'Right, come on Michael, what will we have?' And he'd make him something special.

Mother of Michael (age 8)

It would seem that Michael, who was recognised as having no control over his bed wetting because of his renal problems, had captured the heart of the hotel owner, Dave, as he had won the sympathy and affection of the taxi driver and many members of the local community at home.

By contrast, Sarah's mother suggested that her daughter's bed wetting was not acceptable to others because there was no obvious physical cause for it:

MRS S: I have a urinary problem but people understand that, but then I'm an adult, and I've got MS - that is acceptable. Sarah's is not acceptable to most people ... one friend who we stayed with quite a lot, she'll say 'I would put her in with my daughter but I'm kind of worried in case Sarah has an accident.

Mother of Sarah (age 11)

The effects on the young person's self esteem of other people's negative evaluations of them as a bed wetter are discussed further in Chapter 5. A major determinant of other people's attitudes seems to be the extent to which the young person is perceived as having some control over the situation.

What do parents do of their own volition to encourage the young person's bed wetting to stop?

The methods most commonly used by the families in this study were restricting the young person's fluid intake before bed time, lifting the young person to use the toilet at the parents' own bed time and waking the young person in the night. Almost all parents had also tried to encourage the young person's efforts by using various incentives and many had also punished the young person for bed wetting. None of these methods has a good track record of success and in some cases they may actually hinder the attainment of dry nights.

The results of surveys reported by Devlin (1991), Foxman et al (1986) and Haque et al (1981) support the impression gained in this study, from speaking with health visitors, that many families with a bed wetting child rarely if ever seek help from health care professionals. These families may therefore rely on methods which they devise for themselves, together with the suggestions of wider family and friends, in some cases.

Modification of evening and night time routines

Lifting and waking the young person at the parent's bed time and in the night
With only one exception the parents of all the young people in this study said that, at one time or another, they had tried lifting the young person and taking them to use the toilet at their own bedtime in an attempt to keep the young person from wetting the bed through the night. The most striking finding was that some parents had persisted with this method for anything up to eight years and had only stopped the practice when the child was too heavy to lift. Most parents said that lifting the child did save the occasional wet bed and were thankful when the contents of a full bladder had been voided in the appropriate place:

> MRS S: Sometimes ... you were lucky. It is quite a quantity. We're not talking about a little dribble here, we're talking about a full bladder and that is amazing. You know, I used to think 'Oh, thank goodness that is not going to be in the bed!' (laughs). Mother of Sarah (age 11)

The young person's lack of awareness of events and the extent of their disorientation on being lifted in the night was commented upon by several parents. Some young people were said to be placid but others were decidedly obstreperous and could resist the parent's attempts at waking them:

MRS C: Well, the doctor told me to wake her up at night time to go to the toilet, but she loses her temper with me and she keeps telling me to - says bad words! She doesn't like getting annoyed. She doesn't like getting up.

Mother of Carol (age 17)

Alison's mother had been advised to use an intensive waking schedule. This involved her in setting an alarm at 1½ hour intervals throughout the night. She persisted with the method for two months but the bed wetting had continued:

MRS A: In the end she was going to school tired and greeting (crying) and she was still wetting the bed, and she was tired. ...It ended up that she was tired and I was tired so we gave that up!   Mother of Alison (age 9)

Many parents were persisting with a method which they knew to be of limited value:

MRS L: We lifted two or three times a night, but she still managed to wet. She still managed to wet the bed. We used to lift her but I've even seen us lifting her one night and within ten minutes she's doing the toilet and within ten minutes she's wet.   Mother of Lisa (age 4)

Other mothers also commented that the young person could wet the bed within an hour of being lifted. It was as though these parents were falling back on a habitually used practice and persisting with a method of limited value because they knew of no better way to deal with the situation and had discovered that health care professionals also had a limited repertoire of responses. Several parents did, however, comment on a benefit arising from adopting this strategy. They said that doing something made them feel less helpless than doing nothing, even if what they did do was not particularly effective.

Restricting fluid intake before bed time Restricting a young person's fluid intake after a certain time in the evening is a commonly reported practice among parents (e.g. Bollard and Nettlebeck, 1989; Haque et al, 1981; Butler, 1987). This method was being used by eight families at the time of the study and, with one exception, it had been tried by all the parents in the study at one time or another. As with lifting, some parents had persisted with this method for many years. The parents of seven young people said that restricting the young person's fluid intake had always been their practice.

Most young people were given their last drink at their tea time at around 5-6 p.m. Some mothers even restricted fluid intake at this time. Most young people seemed to have accepted the practice, but perhaps some had not been given very much choice:

> MRS M: He accepts it, he does, he doesn't stand and create for any more. If he did, I wouldn't be giving him it.   Mother of Martin (age 6)

As with lifting, the parents said that they had persisted with the practice of restricting fluid intake at night even when it seemed to make little or no difference to the outcome:

> MRS T: She doesn't get drinks after 6 o'clock ...
> MOYA: And have you always done that?
> MRS T: I've always done that.
> MOYA: And do you find that that makes any difference?
> MRS T: No.   Mother of Tracy   (age 9)

Restricting fluid intake in the evening seems to be another example of parents falling back on a response based on habit, in the absence of knowing of anything more effective to try . Unlike lifting and waking the young person at the parents' own bed time, restricting the young person's fluid intake carries with it potentially harmful side effects (Butler, 1994) and is likely to increase the risk of urinary tract infections as one mother had come to realise for herself:

> MRS S: Well, she would waken up and she'd - 'I've got a sore bottom, its burning' (tearfully). What do you do for that? You give them a lot of liquid! ... So this is something we've had to live with as well. A lot of problems with urinary infections.
>
>   Mother of Sarah (age 11)

Sarah's mother had abandoned fluid restriction after only six months for this reason.

Other methods devised by parents Some parents had devised other methods for themselves. When she thought that the problem could be that her son was sleeping too deeply to wake up to a full bladder, Peter's mother had tried removing some of the bed clothes so that he would sleep more lightly. Carol's mother had thought that her daughter might sleep more lightly in a noisier environment and she had conducted an experiment to test her hypothesis. She moved her daughter into a bedroom at the front of the house:

CAROL: I wondered why the room was cold in the middle of the night when she woke me up. She always opened the window because she kent [knew] the fire engines came past the window. She got up to check me to see if I was awake, and here was me still lying on my bed, the same way, not moved a muscle yet.

MRS C: So that didn't work.   Carol (age 17) and her mother

These experiments are an indication of some parents' attempts to take control in a situation where all the methods suggested by health care professionals had failed. These initiatives, while memorable to the families, were usually short lived and merely punctuated prolonged periods when the only methods that they used were known to them to be of limited usefulness. Parents' lack of success with their own methods was often said to have contributed to their feelings of helplessness. However most parents had not totally given up hope that a solution to the problem would, one day, be forthcoming.

The use of rewards

All parents said that they had used rewards at one time or another as an incentive and this was said to have been the first method tried by some parents. The mother of the twins resorted to the use of rewards when she was told by health care professionals that they could do nothing to help until the boys were seven years old:

MRS J: ... I thought, 'Oh God, I've got to wait to 7!', ken? Then that was when I started myself, like the bribery, the rewards.
                    Mother of John and Stephen (age 8)

She had tried offering sweets, toys, days out and bigger rewards such as a bike or a computer game at Christmas. None of "the bribery" worked and she had found it very difficult to offer the rewards in a consistent way:

MRS J: Half the time I gave in. 'But you said we were to get it'. 'Only if you didn't wet'. 'I didn't wet'. 'Oh, take it!'... I gave in quite a lot, just for peace and quiet.   Mother of John and Stephen (age 8)

Peter's mother had found it difficult to be consistent too, especially when the system of rewards and penalties became rather elaborate:

MRS P: We had a system at one point, and saying, 'Right, we'll give you 50p for each dry night', and it got to the stage that he was quite happy to take the odd 50p he'd get, so the other side of the system that - 'Right, you get 50p when you're dry, and I'll take something off when you're wet'!

MR P: (laughter) So he was in debt! In an overdraft!

MRS P: It just all got very complicated - and you say, you know, 'Well, if you can crack - if you can be dry for a month I'll buy you ..' and I knew I was on a dead bet because he never ever managed it.

> Mother and stepfather of Peter (age 15)

The fact that Peter was "happy to take the odd 50p he'd get" suggests that he had little conscious control over the situation and only achieved the occasional dry night, in spite of the offer of tangible incentives to encourage him to make a special effort.

It was some young people's inability to achieve any dry nights, and the resulting disappointment, which had led the parents of three children to stop the practice of offering rewards altogether:

> MRS L: ... She's getting up in the morning and the first thing is she's looking if she's wet and she's maybe going about with her face tripping on her and we have a wee tear, 'I cannae get'.   Mother of Lisa (age 4)

Simon's mother had also recognised that the offer of a reward, whether by herself or the health visitor, had made the stakes too high and had resulted in Simon hiding his wet night-clothes. She had interpreted this as the sign of his desperation to be dry and his distress at not achieving this goal.

The mothers of Alison, Simon and Lisa discovered from experience that the offer of rewards for dry nights was inappropriate for their children, who were wetting the bed seven nights per week. This has important implications for practice as it may be that the offer of even very small rewards for dry nights is inappropriate for those young people who wet the bed most frequently.

The offer of a large reward for a prolonged period of dry nights, mentioned by several parents, is not only unrealistic and unlikely to be successful as a motivational aid, it is also, effectively, a form of punishment in that an unattainable reward is a privilege withheld:

> MRS T: My mum had taken this boy [Tracy's brother] to America when he was nine, and she says, 'If you stop wetting the bed, Tracy, I'll take you'.
> Mother of Tracy (age 9)

A more subtle form of punishment was hinted at by Sarah's mother when discussing Sarah's motivation to be dry:

MRS S: Well the motivation, if it is strong enough, is to please mum or to please dad, you know, it's not for themselves. Sarah comes to me, her eyes a-twinkle, 'I've not wet the bed tonight, mum'. I say, 'That's brilliant', and she'll give me a big cuddle - she's rewarding me!

Mother of Sarah (age 11)

It would seem that Sarah wanted her mother's approval more than money, bikes or computer games, which were the rewards most commonly offered by parents for dry nights. Sarah's mother had punished her daughter for wetting the bed in the greatest variety of ways reported on in this study. She had used shaming and tirades, physical punishment, withdrawing privileges such as watching favourite TV programmes and threatening to throw away her daughter's clothes. Parents' use of punishment to discourage the young person's bed wetting is now described.

The use of punishment

MOYA: How do you feel about punishing children who wet the bed?
HV A: Well I think that's inappropriate, but I can quite see why people do. I think it would be very easy just to give the child a quick slap round the ear hole, but I don't recommend it and I would certainly frown on it, but I think as a human being I can quite see that I might easily do the same.

Health Visitor A

An analysis of parents' feelings about bed wetting showed that the majority of parents felt frustrated, at times, with what they regarded as a never ending problem. Some parents said that they felt angry with the young person for not making sufficient effort to help themselves to overcome the problem. Parents from two families went so far as to suggest that the young person deliberately wet the bed on some occasions.

When analysing the data about parents' use of punishment there seemed to be a close correlation between parents' negative feelings about bed wetting and the bed wetting child, their perception of the young person's control over the phenomenon and their use of punishment. The use of various forms of verbal and non-verbal punishment has been found in this study to be much more widespread than some of the literature suggests (Chapter 1).

Parents in 13 of the 19 families in this study said that they had punished their child for wetting the bed on some occasions. Five mothers said that they had used physical punishment, especially when they thought that the child was being lazy or when they themselves had felt particularly frustrated:

93

MRS J: Sometimes I would slap her out of sheer anger or frustration .. I used to scream and shout and then that was it.

Mother of Jennifer (age 9)

MRS C: I spanked her. I used to smack her a lot for doing it. Well I used to smack her quite a lot when she started to do it. I used to shout at her and stop her having any sweets and it still didn't work.

Mother of Carol (age 17)

What Carol's mother had not realised at the time was that her daughter was being abused by her natural father when she stayed with him at weekends, after the parents had separated.

Tracy's mother was finding it very difficult to cope alone with four children and she too had used physical punishment until only a few months before the study, when her health visitor had discovered about Tracy's bed wetting when carrying out a developmental check on one of the younger children:

MRS T: I do - I did hit her at first - I used to get up in the morning and hit them - but it was Doreen (health visitor) that spoke to me, she says, 'Don't Ann,' she says, 'I know I'm getting on tae ye, but it's going to make it worse.' She says, 'I understand what you're going through'.

Mother of Tracy (age 9)

In two families a punitive approach was said to have originated from the father but had not had the desired effect of bringing about dry beds. For Gary's parents the difference in their approach to the use of physical punishment had become an issue within the family:

MRS G: We're arguing about it all the time. To hit him willnae solve the problem - to hit him doesnae make any difference. The health visitor says to me, 'You've like got to continually ignore it'. You can only ignore it for so long, and it just boils over, - but I didnae hit him for it. And he thinks he should get hit all the time for it, but I dinnae think so, cos he doesnae know that he's wet the bed at night.

Mother of Gary (age 5)

Encouragement to punish the child physically was said to have come from other family and friends in some cases:

MRS A: My mum ... had the old belief that wetting the bed was 'lazyitis', that skelping her bum would soon stop it, but it didnae work. We just gave her rows, we didnae spank her, we just gave her rows, ken, 'You're dirty',

94

ken, 'This is not on', sort of thing. But it was no' working, so after two or three days we stopped it. That wasnae having any effect.

Mother of Alison (age 9)

Rows, shaming, and shouting at the young person in the morning, on discovering a wet bed, were far more commonly reported than the use of physical punishment:

MRS M: I must admit we used to - did used to get on to him now and again about it, because it got to us. We never never hit him or anything for it because - but we used to really - we were quite firm with him. The odd morning we'd maybe shouted at him a wee bit, but it wasn't his fault. He didn't do it to annoy me or anything, he just couldn't help himself. Just one of these things.

Mother of Martin (age 6)

Four mothers said that they had tried to shame the child into trying to be dry:

MRS T: And I would say to Tracy, 'Look at Kerry Ann, she's a lot younger, she's not even at school', - ken I've tried to put that intae her but she's just no.

Mother of Tracy (age 9)

MRS S: And I try and shame her with this smell. But she's not ashamed of it! We don't have a problem with it.

Mother of Sarah (age 11)

Sarah's mother was concerned that if she took the clinical psychologist's advice and played down the problem Sarah would think that wetting the bed was normal.

In contrast to the above accounts, eight mothers said that they did not believe in punishing a child for bed wetting, although they might punish the young person for other misdemeanours, including daytime wetting when the young person was thought to have some control.

Ten of the 19 mothers in this study had either been a bed wetter themselves or had experience of living with a bed wetting brother or sister (Appendix A). Six of the eight mothers who said that they did not believe in punishment for bed wetting came from this group. Two of these mothers said that in their experience punishment caused needless distress and was ineffective. They gave this as the reason why they had not punished their own child for bed wetting:

MRS J: If they need, like normal behaviour, if they need a skelp [slap] they get a skelp. But not for bed wetting, because you know I went through it and my Dad was hard on us and it never made any difference. Whereas we just felt really bad for wetting the bed and we were feared to say we had wet the bed, because he was quite stern about it and that. Once or twice we got skelped [slapped] for it because none of his were bed wetters, not his brothers or his, ken - just us and we were bed wetters.

Mother of the twins, John and Stephen (age 8)

While some mothers said that they were against the use of punishment because of the adverse effects they had seen it could have, as well as its lack of effectiveness, Shelly's mother said that she would not punish her daughter because she herself had not been punished. Ian's parents felt that he had no control over the bed wetting and that punishment was therefore inappropriate. Simon's mother held a similar view:

MOYA: Have you used any punishments at all?
MRS S: Punishments? No! (sounds astounded)
MOYA: How do you feel about punishment? You sounded aghast.
MRS S: I think that would have worked adversely ... it's too negative, isn't it? You have got to be positive about it. I wouldn't punish.

Mother of Simon (age 8)

What are families' experiences of methods suggested by health care professionals?

This section describes families' experiences with methods suggested by health care professionals to encourage the young person's bed wetting to stop, in particular the use of charts linked to incentives, body worn alarms and medication.

Charting progress and the use of incentives

At one time or another all the young people in this study had recorded their progress towards being reliably dry at night, using some form of chart. Usually incentives were linked to the achievement of one or more dry nights. Various incentive regimes had been suggested to parents by health care professionals including stars and progressively larger rewards for more dry nights. The health care professionals' involvement in this way often formalised an approach which parents had adopted for themselves. Some of the problems associated with the use of rewards to motivate young people to take responsibility for becoming dry are described earlier in this chapter. The present section focuses on family members' experiences with the charts themselves.

Some children were said to have embarked on the use of a chart with optimism and enthusiasm:

> MRS S: He was always excited coming home with his new charts and stars and whatever, weren't you? (to Simon). I think you just got frustrated with them because they weren't working.   Mother of Simon (age 8)

Seven young people were said to have made some progress while they kept a chart:

> MRS G: The psychologist gave me a star chart ... that worked for three weeks, then it was, the novelty wore off for him and there just wasnae any fun in it for him any mair.   Mother of Gary (age 5)

All the parents said that in the end the young person had given up when their progress was not sustained.

For four young people incentive charts were said to have been a cause of disappointment from the start. Stephen's mother described the chart as "useless" and Shelly's mother as "a waste of time". Each of these young people was wetting the bed seven nights per week and could not achieve even one dry night. In sympathy Lisa's mother had given her a star sometimes "for being a good girl":

> MRS L: She knew that it wasn't right [to receive the star], so that went in the bucket.   Mother of Lisa (age 4)

For Peter (age 15) and Sarah (age 11) an important issue had been where to put the chart to avoid their friends coming upon it by chance. Sarah had kept a chart diligently at first but had been put off using it when someone had commented upon it:

> MRS S: 'I'm not having that up on the wall and people will think I'm babyish. It's going away. You don't get stars when you are a big girl, you only get stars when you're in Primary I'. Which is true. Do you ever see stars in anybody's reading book in Primary V and VI? I don't think so.
>   Mother of Sarah (age 11)

The inappropriateness of stars as an incentive was also commented upon by the mothers of Tracy and Martin:

MRS M: He wasn't awfully interested in that, it wasn't something he thought like getting a star at school and that. It didn't do a lot for him.

Mother of Martin (age 6)

Martin and his mother tried the chart for a week. In Tracy's household the method had lasted for two days:

MRS T: She's no' using it - I put it in the first morning to show her, and she put it in on the second one, and that was it. I don't know what she's done with it.   Mother of Tracy (age 9)

Tracy's mother was kept fully occupied looking after four children on her own and she had not managed to find time to keep the diary for this study either.

Charting progress can be a helpful way of demonstrating to the young person that they are capable of achieving dry nights (Blackwell, 1995; Butler, 1993 a,b; 1994):

MR A: Whenever a chart is being kept things have improved. As soon as there's a hands-off approach, there is no physical recording or anything like that, then the whole thing goes haywire.

Father of Anthony (age 16)

Both Anthony and Alison experienced many fewer wet nights during the diary keeping for this study. Alison had found the diary keeping easy:

MRS A: She found it very very easy. She found it great, no trouble at all. She's enjoyed it! ... It worked a lot better than the star charts. The star charts didn't work at all, but that was like she would get a reward if she managed it three days, but she couldn't do that and she didn't take part in it either. I think marking the chart yourself works because she's taking part in it too. She did it all herself.   Mother of Alison (age 9)

Alison's mother made two important observations. She felt that the chart had worked because Alison had taken an active part in keeping it and there had been much less pressure on Alison because the chart had not been linked to any system of tangible rewards. She was praised simply for keeping the record but she also came to see that dry nights were possible. At the end of the month the frequency of Alison's wet nights had fallen from seven to two per week and she wanted more diary forms. It is suggested that the supportive climate created by both Alison's parents had a great deal to do with Alison's success but she could have become dry during this period by chance.

In contrast, the mothers of Martin and Tracy had had little faith in the charts and the record keeping had lasted less than a week. The parents' pivotal role in creating the climate for the young person to learn or re-learn the skill of becoming dry at night is developed further in Chapters 5 and 6.

Bedside and body worn alarms

Fourteen young people in this study had used a body worn alarm at one time or another and four young people were using one at the time of the study. Some parents suggested that the alarm woke everyone on the household except the child and was difficult to switch off. In Anthony's family the alarm had become a family joke, long remembered and used for a very short time. Anthony himself described the alarm as "very tedious".

Several parents commented that the alarm had caused the young person a considerable degree of distress during the night. Jennifer had a clear opinion of the alarm:

> JENNIFER: It's uncomfy. When you went to the toilet you had to take the whole alarm off and put it back on again. It took ages...
> MOYA: So if someone suggested to you that you try it again, what would you say?
> JENNIFER: Get lost!!   Jennifer (age 9)

William began treatment with an alarm during the study. The adverse consequences for everyone in the family were said by his mother to have changed her attitude to his bed wetting:

> MRS W: I feel that our attitudes to his bed wetting had changed because of the buzzer, and it's not improved ... To me, before, it wasn't a problem, and the only reason that I did something about it was for William - it wasn't for me ... now, it's intruding on me as well. And I suppose because I'm back at university and, I'm sort of feeling that I need my sleep - and it's you know - it's irritating me ... My attitude's gone from being very laid back about William to being - well, ... I'm getting up here every night, and I expect to see something, ... - I mean - don't get me wrong, I'm not saying it to him, but it's annoying to me now because it's intruding in my life and because we're not getting anywhere.   Mother of William (age 9)

This is, perhaps, one of the most disturbing findings of families' experiences of an alarm. Not only had this treatment failed to bring about the desired effect, it had also changed the mother's expectations and led her to experience negative feelings, where before she had felt relaxed about the bed wetting.

Few parents in this study had used a body worn alarm for any length of time because of the inconvenience that it had caused to everyone in the household, yet the results of carefully controlled clinical trials (e.g. Butler et al, 1988, 1990; Fordham and Meadow, 1989; Kaplan et al, 1989) suggest that the body worn alarm can achieve a high success rate, when carefully supervised, and has a considerably lower relapse rate than the use of medication alone. The experiences of the families in this study perhaps reflect health care professionals' lack of awareness of the amount of support young people and their families need with a method which requires sustained commitment from the whole family for many weeks to stand a good chance of success (Butler, 1994; Devlin and O'Cathain, 1990; Dische et al, 1983; Fordham and Meadow, 1989; Forsythe and Butler, 1989; Johnsen, 1992; Larsen et al, 1992; Meadow, 1977; Morgan, 1993).

Medication

Half the young people in this study had been prescribed medication for their bed wetting at one time or another. Nine young people had been prescribed Desmospray and five were taking Desmospray at the time of the study. In three cases it had certainly been associated with a dramatic fall in the number of wet nights per week. There is a growing body of evidence in support of Desmospray's efficacy and mode of action (eg. Hjälmås & Bengtsson, 1993; Meadow, 1989; Rittig et al, 1989; Stenberg & Lackgren, 1994). It had not proved so successful for Peter and Sarah but it transpired that both these young people had lost faith in it as a method and only used the spray intermittently:

> MRS S: ... I said, 'You know it seems to be doing quite well, Sarah, you've not been wetting the bed, we seem to be dry quite a lot'. She said, 'It doesn't make any difference whether I take the spray or not'. I said, 'When you take the spray we seem to have had quite a few -'.'But I sometimes don't take it just to see if I'll wet the bed and sometimes I don't wet the bed, so it doesn't work'.   Mother of Sarah (age 11)

There is an important lesson for health care professionals in this account. Young people are not merely passive recipients of advice and cannot be assumed to be complying with the treatment prescribed. They evaluate the methods that they are asked to take part in and may act on their evaluation.

When incentive charts had failed Carol had been prescribed Imipramine, which she had supposedly been taking for the past year and a half. Carol did have some symptoms suggestive of an unstable bladder, which may be the reason why this medication had been prescribed, but the researcher's observation of the tablet bottle suggested that few tablets had been taken in the previous six months. Nothing that Carol had tried had had any lasting beneficial effect for her. Peter had also been prescribed Imipramine but his mother had become concerned that he was becoming dehydrated and he had stopped taking it. Martin's mother had also been concerned about her son taking medication but she had been delighted by the results:

> MRS M: I've never really looked back. It's like a magic potion - it has, from the first night, I can't believe that it could have, it's done the trick.
>
> Mother of Martin (age 6)

Martin was on a reducing dose of Tryptizol and his mother's main concern was that the bed wetting would recommence when he ceased to take it. There is evidence that the beneficial effect of anti-depressants disappears when the drug is discontinued and there is increasing concern being expressed by some clinicians about the use of anti-depressant medication in children (Wille, 1994), although their use is still recommended by some psychiatrists (e.g. Ambrosini, 1993). One of the biggest hazards is accidental poisoning if insufficient care is taken to keep the tablets out of children's reach. Many adverse side effects are also associated with their use (Wille, 1994).

Complementary medicine

The parents of Anthony and Paul had tried complementary medicine in their search for a cure for the young person's bed wetting. Both had tried hypnotherapy, at the suggestion of their local GP, but without any really long-lasting success. Paul had little recollection of what had happened during the hypnotherapy but his mother was sure that it had had some positive benefits. Hypnotherapy has been found to be an effective treatment in some cases (Edwards and van der Spuy, 1985; French, 1992; Simpson, 1991).

Anthony's family recollected the herbal treatment and their involvement in it vividly:

> MRS A: We had to eat pumpkin seeds ...
> SUSAN: Anthony had to do it, and we would say 'We'll eat one if you eat some'.
> MRS A: So we put them on his breakfast cereal, we tried to cook with them, we tried sweets.
> MR A: Pumpkin cakes! (laughs)

MRS A: We tried everything - even today we would go up and in a drawer, in a very obscure place upstairs, we open it up and there are pumpkin seeds and Anthony is now 16! (all laugh). He would say he'd had them, he'd put them down his trousers, they were everywhere ... they're revolting things - so we gave up on that one!

Mother, father, and sister of Anthony (age 16)

It would seem that Anthony was less optimistic about this treatment than the rest of the family and had only participated in it half-heartedly. Anthony's family, like the families of Peter (age 15), Paul (age 13) and Ian (age 13), had made a concerted effort to help the young person to become dry over many years, yet without the reward of a successful outcome.

How do parents evaluate the help received from health care professionals?

Parents clearly had opinions about the help that they had received from health care professionals and articulated these opinions in a quite unsolicited way, for the most part. The parents' comments have important implications for practice.

Questioning the overall attitude and approach of health care professionals

The attitude of some health care professionals had clearly upset some parents:

MRS L: It was their attitude all the way through. It was students and one sort of head doctor -'It's all in her brain, all in her mind' They went to put dye in her, but she wouldn't sit long enough for them to get a good picture ... Any time I mentioned about that she wet maybe two or three times a night, they said, 'It's not smelly anyway' and I said, 'It is!'

Mother of Lisa (age 4)

The medical students had discounted the views of Lisa's mother about the social consequences of bed wetting, such as the smell of the urine, and had embarrassed her with persistent questioning about the sleeping arrangements in the house. This mother was made to feel that she was to blame. Attempting to carry out invasive investigations on a 2½ year old was almost doomed to failure as it is unrealistic to expect a child of this age to be able to co-operate. Such attempts could also lead a child to become frightened of further investigations. The students had been angry because Lisa wouldn't sit still.

102

This particular consultation had obviously been unsatisfactory for everyone. The mothers of Lisa and Sarah had felt that they were being personally blamed for their daughters' bed wetting.

> "MRS S: ... they tend to - they look for a scapegoat. They do do it. You get it the whole time - I get it from Dr D (the paediatrician) even. 'Well, you know, she lives in a high stress house and' ... and I say, 'I don't think it's really that high stressed, is it?' 'Yes, it is'.   Mother of Sarah (age 11)

Four mothers questioned the approach that health care professionals had adopted with their children. In contrast to the excellent relationship that the whole family had with their GP, Jennifer's mother felt that the doctor who had seen her daughter about the bed wetting had not managed to establish a good relationship with her during the consultation:

> MRS J   Jennifer didn't like her and I felt we got off on the wrong foot. I felt Jennifer wasn't at ease with her. Jennifer wouldn't speak to her ... you've got to get on with the kids, relate to them or they clam up and I feel that's what Jennifer was doing.   Mother of Jennifer (age 9)

Because of the embarrassment and shame that most young people feel about their bed wetting Jennifer's reluctance to talk with a stranger about it is not surprising. Such conversations require to be conducted with considerable tact and understanding on the part of the therapist. Jennifer was much more relaxed and talkative when taking part in this study but the conversations were taking place in her own home and at a pace set by the family.

Anthony's parents described how he had become more reliably dry while keeping a chart but that a visit to the hospital had set back progress:

> MRS A: I remember when we stopped the charts. I tell you what stopped the charts! We went to a clinic and it wasn't Dr. P (paediatrician) it was one of his - one of the ladies - and she said to Anthony ..'I'll see you in six weeks time - and you will be dry - I know you'll be dry'... So we did the star charts, and we wet, and we wet, and were wet, and as soon as he was dry, he didn't want to go any more. That was a very significant part, I remember that, and we did ask and it was 'Because that lady said I'd be dry, and I'm not'. So the star chart was a gonner.
>
> Mother of Anthony (age 16)

Anthony himself recalled his disappointment at being told that he would be dry at certain ages and not finding that he was dry when he reached these ages. It could be that the pressure caused by other people's unrealistic expectations and the failure to achieve goals set by others had actually set back progress in Anthony's case.

"They've no more ideas"

Six mothers felt that the health care professionals that they had approached had run out of ideas of ways to help them and had left them, effectively, to cope alone:

> MRS A: We always felt there isn't any real help for a bed wetter, there is nothing. I mean the health visitors give you advice and that, but none of it works.   Mother of Alison (age 9)

> MRS J: She [the doctor] more or less said that it was just one of these things. She said something about getting her urine tested which has never happened. She didn't say would I go and take her or whatever. You were just sort of left.   Mother of Jennifer (age 9)

Other parents also commented on the lack of follow up after a consultation.
Three mothers felt that they were simply being re-offered methods which had not worked in the past:

> MRS P: You'd go to your GP and it was always just 'Well, there's various things you can do, there's buzzers, there's this, there's that'. Well, we've been through all that, and that was it.   Mother of Peter (age 15)

Peter's mother had had the idea of forming a self-help group in case any other mothers had ideas to share which might help her son.
Tracy's mother was unimpressed when the clinical psychologist suggested trying charts again:

> MRS T: She just gave her a star chart. I said, 'But the star chart's no use'. I says, 'She's been on all that'. Then if that doesnae work they were going to put her on a bed alarm, but the bed alarm was no use either...Twice we tried the bed alarm.   Mother of Tracy (age 9)

Some parents felt that a client-centred approach merely put the responsibility back on to them when they did not have enough knowledge of the causes of bed wetting and the treatment options to make an informed decision:

MRS S: ... people are talking to you and saying, 'What do you see is the way forward?' as Miss A [the health visitor] would say to me ...'We've tried this and we've tried this, what do you think?' You don't know what's on the market, so I suggest something that we've tried before. 'We know that, but what do you think is next?' Because you haven't got a little box that you can say 'We know why it started'. You have no point to go from. You don't know where to go. You're going into a blind alley as far as you're concerned.   Mother of Sarah (age 11)

Eight mothers expressed the view that their health visitor had been supportive, in general, but tended to avoid raising the subject of the bed wetting:

MRS G: I feel that Brenda's [health visitor] not really - it's no' that she's no' interested, but she's never asked me - like what dae I dae aboot it to try new things - she's never really spoke aboot it.

Mother of Gary (age 5)

Gary's health visitor was visiting the family to support the mother in the care of her baby, who was only 6 weeks old. She was fully aware of Gary's bed wetting but she did not know how to help the mother to deal with it.

It became apparent from the parents' comments that many health care professionals were at a loss as to how to proceed when certain standard methods had failed to achieve the desired outcome. Some health care professionals were said to have lost interest, others attempted to encourage the family to re-try methods which the family had already lost faith in. This is reminiscent of many parents' own response of falling back on a long practised habit when faced with an ongoing challenge and insufficient responses in their repertoire to meet it.

What happens when everyone runs out of ideas?

MOYA: And what happens when you run out of ideas?
MRS A: (laughter) Do most people try everything?
MR A: The answer is brandy! (laughter)
MRS A: Valium. Endless cups of Earl Grey tea for me and brandy and lemonade for John.   Mother and father of Anthony (age 16)

The pervasive and far reaching consequences of bed wetting, for some families, are described throughout this chapter. When analysing parents' feelings about the young people's bed wetting, parents' frustration and feelings of helplessness were recurring themes. For many parents their inability to help the young person was regarded as the worst thing about the bed wetting:

MRS A: You feel helpless, that's exactly it, you don't know what to do for the best for her. She's wetting the bed, you try everything you get suggested to you, nothing's worked and still the bed wetting goes on.

Mother of Alison (age 9)

An unexpected finding was that parents could come to the stage of feeling that they had run out of options when the young person was as young as 4 years old. Families' experiences of methods suggested by health care professionals were such that many families had come to believe that health care professionals had no more helpful responses in their repertoire than the families had themselves. Sarah's mother went so far as to suggest that some health care professionals plucked ideas out of the air:

MRS S: I try anything that anyone will suggest to me, but I think they have run out of options ... it's a major puzzle ... (A) specialist thought it might be because she was ultra brainy. I don't accept that. I think that's just - I don't think they know so they make something up! (laughs)

Mother of Sarah (age 11)

Several parents commented on their reluctance to share the "shameful" family secret that their child wet the bed when the opportunity presented itself, for instance at a pre-school check. Having been reluctant to involve health care professionals in the first place some parents felt that they were regarded as a nuisance if they went back to health care professionals when their first suggestions failed:

MRS M: I've been to the doctor that many times and it's all through this ... And they think I'm like a hypochondriac! It's just been like trying to get help from somebody because you don't know what to do. I know now they say it's common, but you don't realise it's common till it happens to you. No, you don't. I'm sure there are loads and loads, but you can understand, I've kept it hidden for his sake. And a bit for my sake, because you feel you're a bit of a failure - what have you done wrong?

Mother of Martin (age 6)

Many families come to a point when they feel that there is no more that anyone can do. Those mothers who had wet the bed themselves, or had shared a household with a bed wetting sibling, were often the most philosophical in that they believed, for the most part, that the young person would one day be dry, although they did not know when or how this would happen.

The parents of some of the older participants in this study, such as Carol (age 17), Anthony (age 16), Peter (age 15) and Roger (age 14) said that they felt that they had come to a point where they had done all they could for the young person and had tried to hand the responsibility for dealing with the situation to them:

> MRS P: I don't know ... what line I should now take. We've tried it one way and it's not working, we've ruled out the psychologist, we've ruled out being lazy and the placebos ... whether I just take a back seat now and say, 'Well we've given you all the help available, and it's not my problem any more' - you know - and just let him get on with it ...
>
> Mother of Peter (age 15)

What of the young people themselves upon whom responsibility for dealing with the situation may ultimately be devolved? Do they have any more ideas about how to achieve dry nights than their parents and health care professionals have? This study suggests that they do not. Few of the young people in this study had any ideas about why they wet the bed or when the bed wetting would stop, as is described in Chapter 5.

Having explored every avenue that they believe is open to them it is not surprising that most parents and young people give up searching for a solution, in time. Action occurs at the intersection of intention and opportunity (Broderick, 1993). Without a viable course of action there is no opportunity for taking action to achieve the goal of the young person becoming reliably dry at night and the family is often left to cope with the consequences of bed wetting alone.

Summary

In most families in the present study the management of bed wetting was seen by both parents as a natural extension of the mother's child care role. Most mothers acted as the "orchestrator" of events, co-ordinating the activities of people within the household and those outwith it, such as wider family, friends and health care professionals. Fathers were not, however, without influence and some had become directly involved in the day to day practicalities, either at the request of the mother or because the mother was unavailable, at times, because of paid employment or illness.

Although health care professionals' intentions to be helpful were rarely questioned most parents had come to believe, from experience, that these professionals had little help to offer to resolve the problem, irrespective of the age of the young person. Most parents perceived themselves to be and were, for the most part, left to cope with the situation by themselves.

Two thirds of the young people in this study had been punished, at some time, for wetting the bed and many had to face the censure of their siblings from day to day. Maintaining secrecy outwith the family was high on most young people's agenda, motivated, it seemed, by their fear of disapproval and rejection by others for their lack of ability to perform an "easy" task usually achieved by children of three to four years of age. Some young people denied that even their closest friends knew about the bed wetting. Many were anxious about staying away from home or having friends to stay for fear that their secret would be discovered.

The effects of one young person's bed wetting were not confined to the young person and the principal carer but could impinge upon everyone living within the household, affecting relationships within the family and the nature of the family's social contacts with wider family and friends. However, not all families appeared to be equally concerned about the bedwetting. The negative and pervasive consequences perceived by some parents were at one extreme but important end of a continuum of experience. At the other end of the continuum there were a few parents who regarded the family as unaffected or only minimally affected by the bed wetting. Most families seemed to be at a point somewhere between these two extremes.

The nature, antecedents and consequences of parents' and young people's attitudes towards bed wetting are explored in the next chapter. Understanding the beliefs underpinning the perspectives brought by different family members to situations related to bed wetting helps to explain the differences between family members in their tolerance of it and whether or not the bed wetting is appraised, both individually and collectively, as a cause for concern.

5 The relationship between beliefs, feelings and behaviour, in the context of the family's experience of bed wetting

Family therapists are keenly aware that understanding client metaphors is a key to understanding how client realities are constructed. Client metaphors provide the context of a client family's problems, reflect and create client realities, and limit the ways in which the family comes to terms with its problems ... Family therapists are no different from their clients in that metaphors guide and limit their thinking. The theoretical metaphors used by family therapists contextualise, reflect, and create their therapeutic realities and limit the ways in which they understand client words and actions and come to terms with client problems. Any way of thinking about anything can be useful, but it is always limiting.

Rosenblatt (1994) p.14

Social science draws heavily on metaphors to gain an understanding of and to organise thinking about phenomena, for example family systems theory draws on metaphors from cybernetics. In nursing the concept of "family systems nursing" is being developed (Wright and Leahey 1993, 1994). This conceptualisation draws on systems theory and cybernetics.

In his book *Metaphors of Family Systems Theory,* quoted above, Rosenblatt describes the pivotal importance of therapists understanding the ways in which their clients make sense of their world, if interventions are to be effective. He suggests that clients and their therapists may be seeing situations very differently because they are viewing situations with the help of different conceptual frameworks. The focus of this chapter is on understanding how parents and young people view bed wetting and the relationship between family members' beliefs, feelings and behaviour as they interact with one another from day to day. The chapter begins by describing the final stages of theory generation in this study.

The identification of the core concept of "perceived control"

The phenomenon of "perceived helplessness" was identified as a category early in this study. Individuals who perceived themselves (or others) to be helpless believed that they (or others) were unable to influence the situation, that is they believed that the outcome was not contingent on their (or others') efforts. During analysis it became apparent that perceived helplessness was a widespread phenomenon, linked with many negative emotions, in that:

1 almost all the young people in this study who wet the bed perceived themselves to be helpless to stop it and felt ashamed that they could not achieve an "easy" task that most three year olds could accomplish

2 all the parents spoken to had perceived themselves to be helpless to control the situation, at one time or another, and many said that they had experienced feelings of hopelessness and despair at those times when they had felt most helpless

3 most parents had come to believe, from experience, that the health care professionals to whom they had turned for help were also helpless to influence the situation in a therapeutic way.

Perceived helplessness appeared in many guises in the data and was at first identified as the central phenomenon or core concept in this study.

Conceptual analysis of the phenomenon of perceived helplessness involved going back to the data and asking many questions of it, such as:

a what are the conditions that lead individuals to believe that they are helpless?

b how stable is perceived helplessness over time?

c how do parents and young people respond to a situation when they believe that they are helpless to influence it?

d how do young people and their parents interpret and respond to each other's behaviour when either or both believe themselves to be helpless?

e what are the consequences of perceived helplessness for the young people and their parents?

While perceived helplessness was confirmed as being a commonly experienced phenomenon, it was found that some parents who believed themselves to be helpless to influence the situation at the present time nevertheless felt optimistic that their child would one day be dry, while others were pessimistic that the situation would ever be resolved. Optimism about the future seemed to be a particularly important factor in influencing the individual's present feelings about the bed wetting.

Re-evaluation of the concept of perceived helplessness suggested that the concept was transcended by the concept of "perceived control". This concept helped to explain the variety in the data and was found to be of central importance both for young people and their parents. The relational aspects of perceived control, that is how much control individuals perceived others to have over the situation, was found to be particularly important.

The concept of perceived control features in many ways in later sections of this chapter, which describe parents and young people's beliefs about bed wetting and the consequences of these beliefs when translated into action. It is shown that perceived helplessness, is for the most part, situation-specific, that is specific to situations relating to bed wetting and is a more stable experience for young people than for their parents. Many parents believe that they could control the situation if they could find the means. For the minority of parents and young people perceived helplessness appeared to be a more global experience, affecting other aspects of daily living.

The development of a conceptual model to explore the relationships between beliefs, feelings and behaviour

The terms "conceptual framework", "conceptual model", and "model" are often used synonymously in the research literature and are used synonymously here. They represent a less formal and less well developed mechanism for organising concepts of relevance to a common theme than is provided by theory. Polit and Hungler (1989) suggest that this in no way diminishes their importance or value in the research process in clarifying concepts and their associations, in facilitating the generation of hypotheses to be tested and in revealing other, related areas for inquiry.

From the earliest analysis of data from this study certain beliefs appeared to be potent determinants and predictors of the attitudes and behaviour of the young people who wet the bed and those of their parents. These beliefs included beliefs about the cause of the bed wetting and beliefs about the individual's control over it. Other beliefs which seemed to be influencing the nature of parents' actions including their beliefs about what a "good" parent "should" do and their beliefs about the young person more generally, both as an individual and as a member of the family.

The conceptual model, illustrated at Figure 5.3 (p. 119), was developed to facilitate an understanding of the relationship and interplay between beliefs, feelings and behaviour at an interactional level. The related concepts of beliefs, feelings and behaviour, which constitute the principal components of the model, are first defined and discussed in general terms.

Some components of the model and their temporal relationship

The nature of beliefs The term "belief" is rarely defined in the research literature. When concluding a conceptual analysis of "beliefs" in the context of parent-child interactions, Sigel (1985) noted that there was no accepted psychological definition of belief. The term is noticeably absent from many recent textbooks of psychology, appearing neither in the glossary nor in the index. Perhaps this is because "belief" is a term so commonly used in everyday speech that its meaning is taken for granted, yet it is a term which incorporates many subtleties of meaning.

"Belief" is defined by Hewstone et al (1994, p.445) as:

> Opinion held about an attitude object, i.e. the information, thought or knowledge one has about some person, object or issue.

A detailed philosophical discussion of the inter-relatedness of the concepts of belief, knowledge and truth is beyond the scope of this monograph but a review of the work of Lincoln and Guba (1985), Harvey (1990), Root (1993) and Schwandt (1994) suggests that beliefs are constructs of reality which are particular to the individual. These authors suggest that beliefs are knowledge in that the individual "knows" what he or she holds to be true. Belief is defined in The Chambers Dictionary (1994, p.152) as:

> Conviction of the truth of anything; faith; confidence or trust in a person, etc; an opinion or doctrine believed; intuition, natural judgement ...

This definition implies that not all beliefs are based on evidence but may involve acceptance of an idea, perhaps put forward by a credible person, as an act of faith.

Beliefs may be based on the received wisdom of other authoritative figures such as teachers or parents, or health care professionals, which may or may not reflect the wisdom of the prevailing culture, or they may come from direct experience. Beliefs are usually a synthesis of personal knowledge gained from

112

several sources credible to the individual. Beliefs can incorporate knowledge in the empirical sense of verifiable observations but not all beliefs are or can be based on evidence and not all beliefs are conscious. In this study beliefs are defined as: convictions of the truth of something. They are regarded as personal constructions of reality created by individuals to help them to make sense of their world. Beliefs can vary in their specificity. Some are situation-specific, others are more global.

The organisation of beliefs into schemata "Social cognition" is defined by Baron and Byrne (1994, p.125) as:

> The manner in which individuals interpret, analyze, remember, and use information about the social world.

A key finding of research into social cognition is that an individual's thoughts about the social world are not a mixture of random ideas, knowledge and beliefs. On the contrary Shore (1991) and others suggest that information and knowledge, acquired through experience, are organised into "schemata".

Baron and Byrne (1994, p.121) described schemata as "mental scaffolds" that hold and organise information. Their importance lies in the fact that once they are formed they exert a powerful influence on the aspects of the social world that the individual attends to, the information entered into memory (usually information consistent with the relevant schema) and the information that is later retrieved from memory. Schemata usually include an affective component, that is an emotional element, which arises from a cognitive appraisal of the situation. Baron and Byrne (1994, p.125) define schemata as:

> Organized collections of beliefs and feelings about some aspect of the world ... providing structure for the interpretation and organization of new information we encounter.

Schemata are rather like the conceptual frameworks and theories used by researchers to help them to make sense of their world. They may play a key role in individuals' understanding of others and themselves. Schemata have been implicated in stereotyping and prejudice. Once an individual has acquired a cognitive framework or schema about some social group based for example on an individual's race, gender, sexual orientation or religion, he or she tends to notice information that fits readily into the framework and to remember facts that are consistent with it more readily than facts that are not. As a result the stereotype can become self-confirming. Attitudes can function as schemata (Hewstone et al, 1994). They have a cognitive, an emotional and a behavioural component. Prejudice is an example of an attitude which leads those who hold it to reject the members of some group, based on certain beliefs and expectations about them.

Schemata may be a convenient form of shorthand to help individuals to make sense of a complex social world but they are generalisations and the inaccuracy of the inferences that sometimes result from the holding of a particular schema can have far-reaching social consequences.

Hewstone and Antaki (1994) suggest that there are still issues relating to schemata that require theoretical and empirical attention. Schemata have proved to be difficult to demonstrate. They conclude that people act *as if* they use schemata. They also suggest that researchers in this field have lost sight of the importance of discovering more about the contents of schemata. So far the emphasis has been on uncovering the processes whereby schemata are used.

Based on the researcher's observations during this study it is proposed that parents and young people develop schemata about bed wetting. The components of the schemata that appear to be particularly important as determinants of the individuals' attitudes and behaviour are described later in this chapter. Most are related to perceived control and the perceived appropriateness of the young person's behaviour for his or her age.

The relationship between beliefs and behaviour Sigel (1985, p.346) describes beliefs as important "psychological guides" to action. He suggests (p.369) that the absence of a universally accepted definition of belief should not discourage researchers from pursuing an intuitively reasonable perspective:

> ... much of what we do and how we do it, and the social, political or psychological positions we take, are ... related to what we believe about various aspects of social reality and our place in it.

However plausible the idea is that there is a connection between belief and behaviour, demonstrating a relationship between parents' beliefs, their behaviour and the outcomes for children has not proved to be easy in practice (e.g. Dallos, 1995; Murphey, 1992). Similarly it has not proved easy to show a strong relationship between beliefs and behaviour in research relating to health promotion (e.g. Butterfield, 1990; Bunton et al, 1991). It is now recognised that many factors can intervene to modify the translation of beliefs into behaviour including other competing beliefs and personal priorities (Stahlberg and Frey, 1994).

The nature of feelings Social scientists use an array of terms for "feelings" such as "emotion" and "affect". The terms can be used synonymously. Except when referring to research literature, the term "feelings" is used in this monograph because it is the term most widely used by lay people in relation to their emotions and was the term used by the researcher in conversations with family members of all ages.

The term "emotion" is much more commonly defined and described in the literature on a conceptual level than the term "belief". Bernstein et al (1991, p.A-19) define emotion as:

> An experience that is felt as happening to the self, is generated, in part, by the cognitive appraisal of a situation and is accompanied by both learned and reflexive physical responses.

These authors have identified six features of emotions:

- emotions are experiences - that is they are of themselves neither overt behaviours nor specific thoughts

- emotions are passions not actions - that is they happen to or are suffered by the self

- emotions can be positive or negative - positive emotions are usually desirable to the self, negative emotions are not usually desired by the self

- emotions vary in intensity - using temperature as a metaphor, emotions can be described using such adjectives as cool, lukewarm, and hot

- emotions arise, in part, from a cognitive appraisal of a situation - emotions depend on the individual's interpretation of the situation, they are triggered by the thinking self but are also experienced as happening to the self

- emotions are accompanied by physiological and learned responses - some of the responses are reflexive, such as an increased heart rate, and some are learned.

Throughout this study many negative emotions are described together with the contexts in which they arise. These negative emotions include anger, shame and helplessness.

The relationship between feelings and behaviour A review of the debate in the psychological literature about the relationship between emotion and behaviour is given among others by Ford (1992), Lazarus (1991), Skinner (1995) and Weiner (1992). Ford (1992) describes three components of emotion, namely:

- the neural-psychological - that is the general subjective experience of the emotion

- the physiological - which he describes as a supporting pattern of biological processes, and

- the transactional - which he describes as a pattern of motor and communicative actions designed to facilitate goal attainment.

He suggests that emotions provide a potent mechanism for regulating behaviour in the short term because affective experience has an immediacy to it that is hard for the individual to ignore. He also suggests that while emotions may seem to be ephemeral there is a growing belief among some psychologists that emotions may be at least as influential as cognitive processes as determinants of enduring patterns of behaviour, in the longer term.

While it may be that the transactional components of emotions can be and are consciously suppressed by some parents some of the time and are therefore effectively "hidden" from view, it is suggested that the visible manifestations of a parent's first feelings on encountering a situation related to bed wetting are usually all too easy for anyone in the vicinity to see, including the young person whose behaviour is the subject of those feelings.

The relationship between beliefs, feelings and behaviour In the present study feelings were at first envisaged as being temporally and linearly situated between beliefs and behaviour but the situation may be less clear cut than this. Weiner (1992) suggests three possible temporal arrangements for thoughts, feelings and behaviour. These arrangements are illustrated in Figure 5.1. This researcher's conceptualisation of the situation allows that thoughts may be directly influenced by the experience of feelings, which are themselves evaluated as happening to the self, perhaps leading to reinforcement of or an alteration of the parent's behaviour (Figure 5.2). It is envisaged that the parent evaluates his or her own behaviour and actions as these are in progress as well as evaluating the observable consequences of these actions.

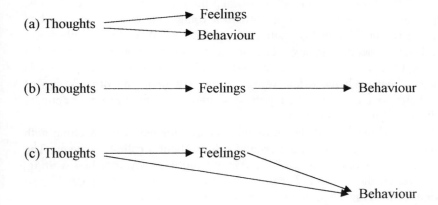

Figure 5.1 Some possible relationships between thoughts, feelings, and behaviour
(from Weiner, 1992, p.363)

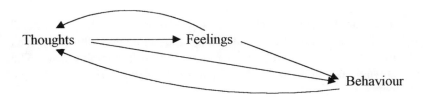

Figure 5.2 An alternative conceptualisation of the relationship between thoughts, feelings and behaviour

Figure 5.3 is a conceptual model illustrating the relationship between beliefs, feelings and behaviour when a parent and a young person who wets the bed interact in (or in relation to) a situation related to bed wetting. It illustrates "mutual simultaneous shaping", one of the central axioms of the naturalist paradigm, being acted out in practice. While acknowledging the uniqueness of the beliefs that each individual brings to any situation, the organisation of beliefs helps to account for the repetitive patterning of the behaviour actually described by family members.

It is proposed that parents come to any situation related to bed wetting with a coherent, organised set of inter-related beliefs about it called a schema. The schema is the cognitive basis of the parent's attitudes towards bed wetting. This collection of beliefs and feelings is based, in part, on the parent's past experiences with this child and perhaps as a former bed wetter.

It is suggested that parents bring many other, more general beliefs to the situation, such as beliefs about:

- self (including beliefs about their capacity to control what happens to them in general)

- being a parent (internalised cultural norms and values about what a "good" parent "should" do)

- the young person, as an individual and as a member of the family.

These beliefs can be conceptualised as being organised into a "system" (Figure 5.4). The term system is used to suggest an integrated whole in which the parts are inter-connected with one another, perhaps in complex ways. The system as a whole is unique to the individual. Each subsystem is a set of topic related beliefs.

It is suggested that beliefs from within and between many sub-systems interact in dynamic, conditional and often predictable ways. Taken together, the beliefs that the parent brings to the situation help to determine the parent's unconscious attitudes and response to the young person's bed wetting and to determine the actions consciously taken.

The schemata constructed by parents about bed wetting are both explanatory and predictive. They help the parent to make sense of what is going on and can help to contribute to the parent's sense of control over the situation. In these ways the parents' schemata are not unlike the theories created by researchers to help them to explain and perhaps predict certain phenomena.

118

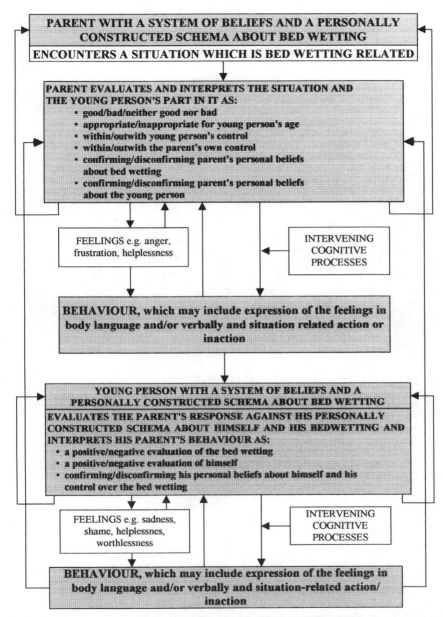

Figure 5.3   A conceptual model of the sequence of events as a
             parent and a young person interpret and respond to
             each other's behaviour during an interaction relating
             to bed wetting

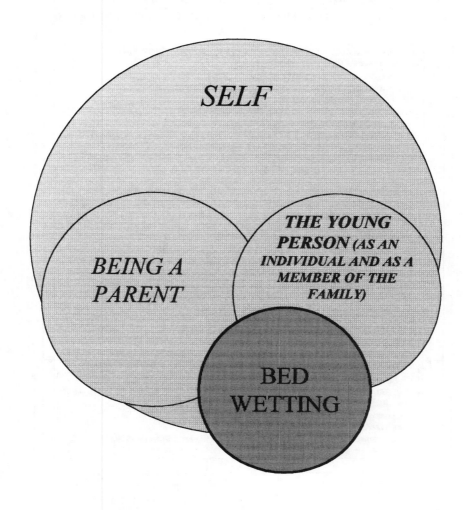

Figure 5.4   **Some components of the parent's belief system**

When a parent encounters a situation related to bed wetting, it is suggested that the parent evaluates and interprets the situation, with the help of the schema, which acts in much the same way as a theoretical lens. It enables the parent to decide almost instantaneously whether the situation is:

- good/bad/neither good nor bad

- appropriate or inappropriate for the young person's age

- within/outwith the young person's control

- within/outwith their own control

- confirmatory or disconfirmatory of their beliefs about bed wetting and about the young person more generally (Figure 5.3).

The parent's bed wetting schema influences those aspects of the situation that the parent attends to, the inferences drawn, and the information that passes into the parent's memory. The parent's cognitive appraisal and interpretation of the situation leads to positive or negative feelings, which may be visibly expressed through body language and may be verbally articulated. The parent's interpretation of the situation also leads to action or inaction. The nature of the parent's action, when taken, may, however, have been modulated by a number of intervening cognitions: such as the perceived priority of bed wetting on the parent's agenda for action ("Do I want to do anything about it just now?"); the anticipation of positive or negative consequences of action or inaction at that moment ("What will happen if I ...?"), and an awareness of the beliefs of other family members and society more generally about what bed wetting is and what a "good" parent "should" do in the circumstances ("What will others think of me if I ...?").

It is suggested that like their parents young people who wet the bed and who find themselves in any situation related to bed wetting, come to the situation with a ready made "system" of beliefs which include beliefs specific to bed wetting and more global beliefs about:

- self

- self, as seen by others

- being a child in this particular family (Figure 5.5).

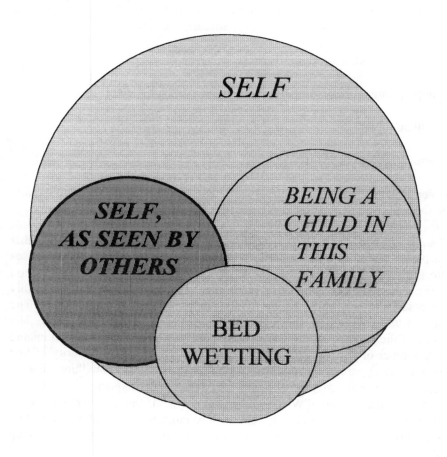

Figure 5.5   **Some components of the young person's belief system**

The young person evaluates the parent's response to the situation in relation to his personal schemata about himself as a person and himself as a bed wetter. He interprets his parent's behaviour as a positive or negative evaluation of himself and as confirmatory or disconfirmatory of his own beliefs about himself and his control over the bed wetting.

It is suggested that beliefs can be changed at any time as a result of a re-evaluation of the situation, but that in reality beliefs about bed wetting are often tenaciously held, in spite of contradictory evidence, which may be "explained" with the help of an elaboration of the individual's personal schema.

It is further suggested that when parents and young people interact and respond to each other's behaviour time after time, perhaps over many years, each individual may for the most part merely be seeing what he or she expects to see. This reaffirms the individual's personal beliefs about bed wetting and the other family members' control over it. This may or may not be helpful for a resolution of the situation in the longer term. It depends very much upon what the contents of the family members' schemata are.

The model's limitations

In this study beliefs have come to be recognised as important determinants of behaviour but it is accepted that the relationship between beliefs, feelings and behaviour is likely to be much more complex than Figure 5.3 suggests. In this study a number of intervening conditions have been identified which seem to be influencing people's choices and actions. It is acknowledged that many factors determine purposeful and unconsciously motivated behaviour and that it is highly probable that in any given situation these factors are interacting in complex ways.

The focus of this study has been on the beliefs brought to situations relating to bed wetting by different family members. These beliefs can be regarded as the "contents" of the psychic system (Leyens and Codol, 1994, p.91). No attempt has been made to explore the cognitive processes whereby information coming from the experience of relating to others, from memory and directly from the senses is received, selected, transformed and built into personal "knowledge", and organised into a schema. This is outwith the scope of this study.

A discussion of the influence of the individual's personality on their evaluation and interpretation of events is barely touched upon, yet it could be an important contributory factor. A discussion of the limits of family members' influence and the interplay between nature and nurture, as determinants of parents' and young people's responses to bed wetting, is also beyond the scope of this monograph. A general discussion of these issues can be found, for instance, in Plomin and Daniels (1987), Plomin (1994) and Rowe (1994).

The present study merely illuminates some aspects of a complex reality.

The application of the model

Analysis of data from this study has led to a greater understanding of the nature of lay beliefs about bed wetting held by family members where one member is a bed wetter and of the consequences which may arise when certain beliefs are held.

Parents' beliefs and attitudes towards bed wetting are shown to have powerful emotional and social consequences for themselves and their children and to help to determine the supportiveness or otherwise of the emotional climate within the home in which the young person is trying (or not trying) to learn the skill of becoming reliably dry at night.

Parents' beliefs about the causes of bed wetting

The beliefs of the parents in this study about the possible causes of their child's bed wetting are summarised in Table 5.1. They can be broadly subdivided into three categories: physiological problems; psychological attributes of the young person, or the young person's response to a negatively perceived event within or outwith the family. These findings are broadly similar to the findings of Haque et al (1981) and Butler and Brewin (1986).

In a survey of 1,435 parents of children consecutively referred to the paediatric department of one of nine medical centres in the United States, Haque et al (1981) found that more than one third of the parents of both bed wetters and non bed wetting children believed that bed wetting had an emotional cause. Parents of bed wetters were more likely than the parents of non bed wetters to attribute the cause to deep sleep and were more likely to attribute it to a condition which ran in families. This may be a reflection of the parents' own personal experience of bed wetting in some cases.

In Butler and Brewin's (1986) study heavy or deep sleep was easily the most endorsed cause of bed wetting by parents, followed by two attributes of the young person as a "worrier" or "easily upset". With the exception of deep sleep, physiological problems tended to be regarded as less significant than psychological causes by the parents in the present study and in the two studies reported above. This runs counter to many health care professionals' belief that bed wetting is primarily a pathophysiological problem (Chapter 1).

124

Table 5.1

Parents' beliefs about the causes of bed wetting

PHYSIOLOGICAL CAUSE	PSYCHOLOGICAL CAUSE	
	AN ATTRIBUTE OF THE YOUNG PERSON	THE YOUNG PERSON'S RESPONSE TO AN EVENT WITHIN OR OUTWITH THE FAMILY
deep sleep	laziness	marital conflict
a problem with the "plumbing" (e.g. small bladder)	attention seeking	parents separating
puberty (e.g. hormonal)	mood at bed time	mother going in to hospital
when ill	"in his mind"	death of the father
	still to learn how	poor relationship with father
		child abuse
		sibling rivalry
		arrival of a new baby
		watching a frightening film
		worried about "something" (cause unknown)

The studies of Haque et al (1981) and Butler and Brewin (1986) do not indicate which parents hold which attributional beliefs and with what consequences. It was found in the present study that the parents' attributional beliefs were on some occasions the basis of methods that some parents tried for themselves to encourage the bed wetting to stop (Chapter 4). These beliefs did not, however, by themselves, seem to account for parents' different attitudes to their child's bed wetting, which are now described.

Parents' attitudes towards bed wetting

There are many definitions of attitude in the literature. Bernstein et al (1991, p.A-14) define "attitude" as:

A predisposition toward a particular cognitive, emotional, or behavioural reaction to an object, individual, group, situation, or action.

Baron and Byrne (1994, p.129) suggest that attitudes involve associations between attitude "objects" (that is any aspects of the social world) and evaluations of those objects, and define attitudes as:

... evaluations of various objects that are stored in memory.

An attitude can be thought of as a personal perspective or viewpoint about something and it has three components: a cognitive component, based on beliefs which are organised into schemata; an emotional component, arising from an evaluation of something as desirable or undesirable, and a behavioural component, that is a relatively stable and enduring way of acting toward the object of the attitude (Stahlberg and Frey, 1994).

A classification of parents' attitudes towards bed wetting

From talking with parents in this study four factors have been found to be particularly important as determinants of behaviour. Certain combinations of these beliefs have been found to be strongly predictive of: a parent's overall attitude to the young person's bed wetting; their behaviour towards the young person, and the emotional and social consequences of that behaviour for the young person and themselves. The factors found to be important are:

- the parents' definition of the bed wetting as appropriate or inappropriate for the young person's age

126

- the extent to which the bed wetting is regarded as a cause for concern

- the parents' beliefs about the young person's capacity to control the bed wetting

- the parents' beliefs in their own capacity to influence the situation at the present time and in the future.

It is suggested that the parent's attitude to his or her child's bed wetting can be classified into one of three broad categories: acceptance and tolerance; ambivalence, or rejection and intolerance. Two of these categories have been further subdivided according to the parents' optimism about the young person becoming reliably dry at night in the future.

Using Strauss and Corbin's (1990) axial coding paradigm as a framework the causal conditions, intervening conditions, interactional strategies and consequences of these attitudes are summarised, in general terms, in Table 5.2. The causal conditions form part of the parent's schema about bed wetting.

Before describing each of these attitudes and their consequences in more detail, it is important to make some general points.

The seven attitudes described are not regarded as personality traits, in the way for instance that Butler et al (1986, 1990, 1993) has used the term "maternal intolerance" to imply a stable trait of the mother. Rather, these seven attitudes are regarded as differing perspectives which parents bring to any situation relating to bed wetting at a point in time, based on certain beliefs held at that time, which give rise to certain general consequences, influenced in practice by many intervening conditions.

These attitudes are not regarded as stable or necessarily consistently held over time. Some of the ways in which these perspectives are thought to change over time are illustrated in Figure 5.6. It is suggested, that even within a short period of time, a parent can vacillate between two of these "positions", for instance between ambivalence and rejection. Some patterns did, however, appear to be more ingrained, for example resigned pragmatic acceptance and tolerance, and resigned rejection and intolerance. While optimistic pragmatism appeared to be the predominant attitude of over half the mothers in this study it is important to emphasise that at least half of these mothers had come to this position from an attitude of rejection and intolerance which had been a relatively stable attitude for them until they had come to believe that the young person could not control the situation. Following definition of the broad categories of: acceptance and tolerance; ambivalence, and rejection and intolerance; each of the attitudes, summarised in Table 5.2, is described with illustrations from parents' accounts of their beliefs, feelings and behaviour.

Table 5.2
Parents' attitudes and responses to their child's bed wetting; causal conditions, intervening conditions, interactional strategies and consequences

(The structure of this table is based on Strauss and Corbin's (1990) axial coding paradigm)

| | PARENT'S ATTITUDE | | | | | | |
| | ACCEPTANCE AND TOLERANCE | | | | AMBIVA-LENCE | REJECTION AND INTOLERANCE | |
	Primary unconditional	Trans-itional	Resigned pragmatic	Optimistic pragmatic		Pro-active	Resigned reactive
A. CAUSAL CONDITIONS							
1. Bed wetting is defined by the parent as appropriate for the young person's age	Yes	Yes	No	No	No	No	No
2. The parent is concerned that the young person still wets the bed	No	Yes, to some extent	Yes	Yes, to varying extents	Yes	Yes	Yes
3. Parent believes that the bed wetting is within the young person's control	No	Not completely	No	No	Perhaps	Yes	Yes
4. Parent believes that he/she has:							
a. the capacity to influence the situation now	No	Yes	No	Yes, in some ways	Perhaps, in some ways	Yes	No
b. the capacity to influence the situation in the future	Yes	Yes	No	Yes	Probably, yes	Yes	No

Table 5.2 continued

	PARENT'S ATTITUDE						
	ACCEPTANCE AND TOLERANCE				AMBIVALENCE	REJECTION AND INTOLERANCE	
	Primary unconditional	Transitional	Resigned pragmatic	Optimistic pragmatic		Proactive	Resigned reactive
B. PHENOMENON Parent's overall attitude to the young person's bed wetting	Parent accepts and tolerates a situation which he/she believes:				Parent has mixed feelings about a situation which he/she believes can probably only be changed by the young person	Parent does not accept and is not prepared to tolerate a situation that he/she believes can be changed:	
	cannot be changed now, but will change in time	should change soon	cannot, or is unlikely ever to change	could change soon		primarily by the young person	only by the young person
C. INTERVENING CONDITIONS 1. Parent's beliefs and feelings about: a) parenting eg the appropriateness/inappropriateness of the use of physical punishment to discourage unacceptable behaviour b) the young person as an individual and as a member of the family c) the quality of their relationship with the young person more generally 2. The priority of bed wetting on the parent's agenda for action 3. The attitude of the parent's spouse or partner, wider family and friends to the young person's bed wetting							
D. INTERACTIONAL STRATEGIES The form that these take depends on the intervening conditions and their interactions 1. Parent takes responsibility for helping the young person to learn the skill of being dry at night	Yes	Yes	No	Yes	Yes	Yes	No

Table 5.2 continued

	PARENT'S ATTITUDE						
	ACCEPTANCE AND TOLERANCE				AMBIVA-LENCE	REJECTION AND INTOLERANCE	
	Primary unconditional	Trans-itional	Resigned pragmatic	Optimistic pragmatic		Pro-active	Resigned reactive
D. INTERACTIONAL STRATEGIES (continued) 2. Parent blames young person on those occasions when he/she loses night time bladder control	No	No	No	No	Yes, sometimes	Yes	Yes
E1. CONSEQUENCES FOR YOUNG PERSON The emotional and social environment for learning to be dry at night (if this is possible) is supportive	Yes	Yes	Yes	Yes	Mixed	No	No
E2. CONSEQUENCES FOR PARENT In relation to bed wetting, feelings of: a) anger towards the young person	No	No	No	No	Yes, sometimes	Yes, often	Yes, very often
b) frustration at the situation	Perhaps	Perhaps	Yes	Perhaps	Yes	Yes	Yes

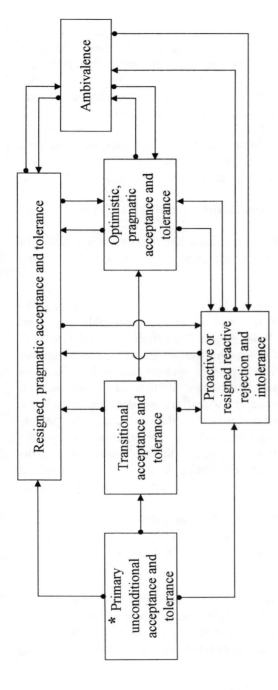

Notes:

* The parent may take any one of many routes originating from an attitude of primary unconditional acceptance and tolerance of lack of

• The parent re-evaluates the situation (perhaps aspects of the situation have changed) and adopts a different attitude to the young person's bed wetting. The change may be sudden or gradual. The changes can occur at any time along the young person's developmental path. The sequencing indicated corresponds to the sequencing suggested by the data from this study, but other sequences are possible.

Figure 5.6 Parents' changing attitudes to the young person's bed wetting (see also Table 5.2)

Acceptance and tolerance are inter-related constructs with several shades of meaning. "To accept" is defined in The Chambers Dictionary (1994, p.9) as:

> ... to take (something offered); to receive (with approbation, favour, consent, resignation or passivity) ...to view favourably or to tolerate ...

While it is unlikely that parents welcome their child's lack of night time bladder control with "approbation" or "favour" some parents seem to consent to it unconditionally, others to tolerate it and others to be resigned to it.

Tolerance is defined in The Chambers Dictionary (1994, p.1821) as:

> ... the ability to resist or endure pain or hardship; the disposition, ability or willingness to be fair towards and accepting of different ... beliefs and opinions; ...

Tolerance suggests a tendency to endure something which may not be pleasant and to treat others fairly, that is justly, reasonably and with forbearance. The definition of "tolerant" as " ...capable of enduring (e.g. unfavourable conditions...) without showing serious effects ..." adds another shade of meaning. It is suggested that parents who are able to be tolerant of their child's bed wetting experience fewer negative emotions in relation to it. Certainly those moments of frustration which are experienced by tolerant parents seem to be less pervasive and persistent than is the case for parents whose overall attitude is ambivalent or intolerant. For accepting parents the frustrations were largely related to the practical difficulties associated with the management of the consequences of bed wetting such as the wet sheets and perhaps the wet child rather than a negative evaluation of the young person as a bed wetter.

Acceptance is a word which describes both an attitude (which has emotional and behavioural components) and a feeling. Ford (1992, p.149) describes the way in which "acceptance", which he groups with affection and love, can help to maintain social relationships:

> The emotion of *acceptance - affection - love* facilitates co-operative social functioning, the development of satisfying interpersonal relationships, and the sheltering and nourishing of helpless persons by supporting the process of interpersonal bonding and the development of mutual commitment and trust between people.

He suggests that this emotion is associated with caring, sharing and service to others and sends the message to the object of the emotion: "We're all in this together".

As is illustrated in Table 5.2, all the parents whose overall attitude towards the young person's bed wetting is one of acceptance and tolerance believe that the young person cannot yet control his or her bladder functioning at night. In this sense the parent regards the child as helpless and is prepared to help him or her to learn to be dry at night, unless it is known that the acquisition of night time continence can never be achieved for pathological reasons. The principal differences that parents within this broad category bring to any situation related to bed wetting are their different beliefs about their own capacity to influence the situation in a positive way (now, or in the future) and their beliefs about the appropriateness of the bed wetting for the young person's age. The four sub-categories of the attitude of acceptance and tolerance are described below.

Primary unconditional acceptance and tolerance Primary unconditional acceptance and tolerance is defined as acceptance and tolerance of a situation that the parent believes cannot be changed now but will change in time. This attitude is described as primary and unconditional in that all (or almost all) parents begin with this attitude when the child is born and maintain this stance for the first few months of the child's life and perhaps for much longer.

During this period parents define lack of bladder control as appropriate for the child's age and they are therefore not concerned about it because the collective wisdom within their local community and the wider society in which they live is that being dry at night is a skill which children are not born with and which they learn in time. The child is not blamed for the lack of control although the parents may feel frustrated from time to time with having to deal with the practical consequences of wet nappies, and perhaps a wet bed.

Transitional acceptance and tolerance Transitional acceptance and tolerance is defined as acceptance and tolerance of a situation which parents expect will change soon. This attitude is described as transitional in that the parents regard the child's lack of night time control as a stage which the child will shortly move beyond. The parents' behaviour is facilitative. The infant is still regarded as a "learner" and parents are usually prepared to tolerate "accidents" during the stage of the learning process when attempts are made to establish control without containment, that is when the child is taken out of nappies on an experimental basis. The parents may feel frustrated if their child appears to be a slow learner, compared to other children of a similar age in the neighbourhood. This raises the question: "At what age do parents begin to become concerned about a child's lack of night time continence?"

In the present study, contrary to many health care professionals' definitions of bed wetting (Chapter 1) most parents said that they had become concerned about the bed wetting some time before the child was of school age.

The survey conducted by Haque et al (1981) found that the mean expected age for attaining night time bladder control was 3.18 years for the 346 parents of bed wetters, compared with 2.61 years for the 1033 parents of non-bed wetting children. It is not known from Haque's study whether the parents who set a higher age for the attainment of dryness had been bed wetters themselves (whether or not their child was a bed wetter) and had learned from experience that achieving night time dryness before the age of 4 years is not always possible.

In the present study six mothers said that they themselves had wet the bed until the ages of 5, 6, 10, 11, 15 and 18 years. With only one exception these mothers were still concerned that their child was not dry before going to school but several stated that their concern was because of the attitude of other people should the discovery be made rather than their own expectation that the child should be dry.

Resigned pragmatic acceptance and tolerance Resigned pragmatic acceptance and tolerance is defined as acceptance and tolerance of a situation which the parent believes cannot, or is highly unlikely to change. This attitude is described as pragmatic and resigned because the parents have realistically given up hope that the situation can be changed, in the light of medical evidence that the young person has an incurable pathological problem or the evidence from their own experience that nothing that they have done has made a difference and the expectancy is that there is nothing more that can be done.

The parent does not actively try to teach the young person to be dry at night but neither is the young person consistently blamed for loss of night time bladder control. The parent may frequently feel frustrated and at times despairing about a situation which is regarded as "never ending". The parents may be angry on occasion with the young person but this is said to be because the young person is not taking sufficient responsibility for those tasks which are within his or her control, such as managing the practical consequences of the incontinent episodes. In the present study there were three clear examples where this attitude was or had been consistently in evidence.

Michael (age 8) was the only young person in this study for whom the cause of the bed wetting was known with any certainty. Michael's mother had to get up to him twice a night on average to change his wet nappy and she had had this to contend with since Michael was born. He also had problems with day wetting. Both Michael's parents were stoical about it but his mother did feel worn down by the constant need to change Michael night and day. She was most frustrated when Michael seemed unaware that he had wet himself:

> MRS M: But - he will go about wet, I keep saying, you know - 'you're not getting a row for being wet, but you're getting a row for going about like that', you know - and I find that difficult to cope with.
>
> Mother of Michael (age 8)

For both parents, however, the predominant concern was that Michael would be hurt by the comments of other people. The frustration that both parents felt at times was openly acknowledged within the family and Michael could actually make a joke about it:

> MOYA: So what's the worst thing about it, about being wet, do you think?
> MICHAEL: Um ... (pause)
> MRS M: Mummy being at you all the time!
> MICHAEL: Yes (laughs). Thank you for saying that, Mum, you've had a brain wave!
> Michael (age 8) and his mother

Michael was such a cheerful child. He seemed to have everybody's sympathy from the taxi driver who took him to school to relatives and friends who took him to watch football because he clearly could not help wetting himself and indeed he was seen to be suffering as a result of his chronic health problem. Michael's father summed up the parents' feelings about Michael's bed wetting:

> MR M: I sometimes think - we maybe try to protect him too much. Up until, especially up 'til he went to school, I think we sort of done everything for him and helped him every way we could, and then when he went to school we started telling him to do things ... 'Come on, you're getting big now, you should be able to realise that this is happening'. And he comes back with an answer like, 'Do you not know I've got a kidney problem?' (Everybody laughs) And you sort of say to yourself, 'God, I know you've got a kidney problem!' He just comes back with these one or two liners - he's quite a character... Sometimes you could murder him and other times, you know, he breaks your heart.
> Father of Michael (age 8)

Although it was a "never ending thing" which continually made both physical and mental demands on them, Michael's parents had come to an acceptance of the situation which they believed they could not change and which was helped when the burden that they were bearing was seen to be recognised by others, for instance when Michael's mother was given an attendance allowance:

> MRS M: ... you feel as if somebody's patting you on the back and saying, 'you know, that's fair enough'.   Mother of Michael (age 8)

Two other mothers, those of Alison (age 9) and Carol (age 17) had also come to an attitude of resigned pragmatic acceptance and tolerance of a situation which both felt unable to influence. This attitude can be summarised as "giving up":

> MRS A: ... you feel helpless, that's exactly it. You don't know what to do for the best for her. She's wetting the bed, you try everything you get suggested to you, nothing's worked and still the bed wetting goes on. You think, the older she gets, it's never going to end ... It's just total despair. We gave up, you know. Leave it, ignore it, we've done everything else, it can't get any worse. We thought we were going to be doomed for the rest of our days to have her as a bed wetter.   Mother of Alison (age 9)

After seven years of unsuccessful attempts to help her daughter to be dry at night Alison's mother had made the conscious decision to stop actively attempting treatments which were patently not working for her. She described the way in which everyone's spirits in the household had improved once the decision was made to do nothing. Before this level of acceptance and tolerance was reached Alison's mother had punished her daughter for the bed wetting when she believed that her daughter had more control over the situation than she was choosing to exercise. Adopting an attitude of resigned acceptance and tolerance does not mean that the parents do not wish that the situation was different. It is merely an acknowledgement by them that nothing more can realistically be done, accompanied by a decision to make the best of the situation that they find themselves in. As such its purpose is one of damage limitation.

The mother of Carol (age 17) had also come to the stance of resigned pragmatic acceptance and tolerance of a situation which she believed was unlikely to change or at least to be within her control. Carol's mother had wet the bed herself until the age of 16 and Carol's father had wet the bed until he was 24 years old so perhaps the expectancy was that Carol would wet the bed into adulthood. Carol's mother and her new partner were not angry about the bed wetting itself, but at Carol's lack of motivation to help herself on those mornings when she did wake up wet.

Optimistic pragmatic acceptance and tolerance This attitude is defined as acceptance and tolerance of a situation which the parent believes could soon change for the better. This attitude is described as optimistic and pragmatic because the parent is hopeful and perhaps confident that the young person will attain night time bladder control in the future but takes a realistic view in the meantime, recognising that the attainment of night time bladder control is not easy for some young people.

These parents believe that they are able to influence the situation in a positive way to some extent but that they may not currently have the means to do so. They take responsibility for helping the young person to learn the skill of being dry at night. They do not blame the young person on those occasions when night time bladder control is lost, but they may feel frustrated by the consequences of the bed wetting such as the extra laundry. The message which they convey to the young person is: "Bed wetting is something which happens to some people, you can't help it and you will grow out of it". These parents are often particularly empathetic towards the young person and express the concern that the bed wetting is stopping them from doing so many things.

In this study five of the parents who had adopted the attitude of optimistic pragmatism were known to have had experience of bed wetting as a bed wetter themselves or from having lived at close hand with a bed wetting sibling. These parents were quite unequivocal that the young person could not help wetting the bed:

> MRS I: I used to try that hard, you know. So I understand how he feels when he's dry for maybe a week and then he's right down in the mouth. I understand how I felt, so I can understand how he feels. It was really disappointing because he thought, 'this is it, I'm dry' - and then the next time you're back again, wetting again. I understand how he feels. Every time he thinks, 'this time,' and I say to him, 'keep your fingers crossed, maybe this is it', you know. Mother of Ian (age 13)

In these families the impression was clearly gained that the attitude of optimistic pragmatism had been consistently held over many years. The young person had never been punished for bed wetting, indeed the parents in each of these families said that they felt that the use of punishment would have been quite inappropriate. In at least four other families, however, parents whose current attitude seemed to be one of optimistic pragmatism, indicated that there had been a time when they had been far less tolerant of the situation. This had been when they had felt that the young person had more control over the bed wetting which they were choosing not to exercise.

Ambivalence is defined in The Chambers Dictionary (1994, p.48) as:

> Co-existence in one person of opposing emotional attitudes towards the same object

Parents with an ambivalent attitude towards their child's bed wetting have mixed feelings about a situation which they believe can probably only be changed by the young person in the end. They believe that the young person may have more control over the situation than he or she is choosing to exercise yet at the same time they are perplexed that the young person does not exercise the control that they may have to combat the negative social consequences of bed wetting.

These parents see their role as encouraging the young person to take responsibility for the situation for themselves and may go to some lengths to find the means to help the young person to achieve dry nights. They may blame the young person on those occasions when night time bladder control is lost and they become frustrated and at times angered by the young person's apparent lack of effort to help him or herself. They are also frustrated in those cases when the young person does not appear to be willing to play a part in the management of those consequences of bed wetting over which they could have some control. However, these parents tend to have a good relationship with the young person on the whole and to have encouraged the young person to pursue interests which give them the opportunity to experience success. These young people therefore tend to be sent a mixed message: "Overall you're OK, but the bed wetting is something which you should be able to control by now, and it is something which you could control if you made more of an effort to help yourself. When you want to, you will be dry."

Many parents may experience ambivalence about their child's bed wetting from time to time but in this study ambivalence was found to be a persistent attitude amongst the parents of some older bed wetters, where the parents felt that all the treatment options had been exhausted. In two cases the mothers expressed ambivalence in the face of their husbands' unequivocally stated belief that the young person could help themselves if they made more effort:

MRS A: But what 16 year old would want to wet the bed every night?
SUSAN: No, but he doesn't really really want it, [to be dry] does he?
MRS A: Why? I could understand when he was tiny, and they used to say to us, OK, he likes the effect of a wet nappy round him. As a little toddler I can understand that, but a 16 year old boy - I mean, come on!! - at 16 years

of age, nearly 17 - he's a young man. His thoughts are of young girls, and of dirty magazines and all that sort of thing that that age group go in for.
MR A: (coughs) I personally believe that will be the point at which the problem will go away.   Mother, sister and father of Anthony (age 16)

The attitude of Anthony's sister Susan is suggestive of sibling rivalry. The mothers of Anthony (age 16) and Peter (age 15) were, however, wanting to give their sons the benefit of the doubt, even when all the evidence seemed to be that the young person was not making as much effort as they could be making to help themselves. It seemed to be a manifestation of maternal protectiveness. In both cases the management of bed wetting was just one item of contention in a catalogue of others, relating to life with an adolescent.

For ambivalent parents, their inability, over many years, to exercise effective control over a situation where they believed that some control was possible had led to feelings of frustration and despair. In each case, however, the young person seemed to be the principal focus of the parents' concern:

MRS P: It's just that you feel so frustrated that you can't help them ... You know the health visitor says, 'Yes, it must be awfully hard having all these sheets to wash', but you get used to it. You know you don't see it as extra work, you feel more sorry for them because it's causing them a problem, embarrassment, whatnot.   Mother of Peter (age 15)

The negative consequences for the family as a social unit are described in Chapter 4. The consequences for the mothers were said to be pervasive:

MRS A: It's frustration ... your whole life - because you always go to bed - wherever you go, whatever you do, it's on your mind ... I'm perhaps menopausal - you're frustrated, you're annoyed, you're hyper, you get PMT, you're a mother, you've had an argument with your husband, and you know - the shopping - it's the thing that comes back all the time, for ever.
                    Mother of Anthony (age 16)

It was a chance conversation with Anthony's mother which influenced the researcher to embark on this study.

Rejection and intolerance

Rejection and intolerance are inter-related constructs and are the converse of acceptance and tolerance. To reject is defined as:

... to throw away; to discard; to refuse to accept, admit or accede to; to refuse; to renounce.   The Chambers Dictionary (1994) p.1452

As a noun a "reject" is defined as: "... an imperfect article ...".

Intolerance is defined as:

> ... not able or willing to endure; ... persecuting; easily irritated or angered by the faults of others ... (p.878)

Parents who are intolerant of their child's bed wetting all have one belief in common. They believe that the bed wetting is within the young person's control. These parents are not prepared to accept and are disinclined to endure a situation which they believe can be changed but ultimately only by the young person. These parents experience feelings of frustration and anger in relation to the bed wetting. The parents who perceive themselves to be least able to influence the situation seem to experience these negative emotions particularly pervasively.

Parents within this broad category differ in two important respects:

1   the extent to which they believe that they are in control of their lives in general (which differentiates between the proactive and the reactive parents), and

2   their feelings of benevolence towards the young person in general, that is the extent to which their rejection and intolerance is situation-specific.

All these parents have a tendency to blame the young person on those occasions when he or she loses night time bladder control and tend not to provide a particularly supportive emotional climate for the young person to learn the skill of becoming dry at night.

Where the intolerance is situation-specific the message sent to the young person seems to be: "Overall you are OK but in relation to the bed wetting you could act differently and you are not helping yourself". Where the intolerance is more generalised the message appears to be: "Overall you are not OK and in relation to the bed wetting you could act differently and you are disobeying my wishes." The two subcategories of the attitude of rejection and intolerance are now described.

Proactive rejection and intolerance Proactive rejection and intolerance is defined as rejection and intolerance of a situation which the parent believes is largely within the young person's control. This attitude is described as proactive because these parents still believe that they have a role to play in encouraging the young person to take responsibility for stopping the bed wetting and in helping the young person to find the means to do so. These parents take the initiative, they actively seek new treatments and try to encourage the young person to persist with them. They follow up new treatment ideas which they come upon by chance, for instance through the media. They are determined to resolve the problem of the bed wetting. They may or may not exhibit benevolence towards the young person more generally.

The fathers of Anthony (age 16) and Peter (age 15) fall into this category. Both appeared to be benevolent towards their sons in many ways. Benevolence is a disposition to do good, to act out of kindness and with generosity. These parents seemed to be well disposed towards their children in general but they clearly disapproved of the bed wetting. Their rejection and intolerance is therefore seen to be situation-specific.

Having run out of physical explanations these fathers had come to what seemed to them to be the logical conclusion that the problem was a psychological one and therefore within the young person's control:

MR P: Well, I'm no doctor, but maybe I'm wrong - but I think you've basically got two sides. You've got the plumbing side with the urologist, then you've got the psychological side. Now if the plumbing side is all right, it's either the chemistry of the body somehow or the psychological side. Once you can rule out these two points it's a matter of, in my opinion you've got to re-educate Peter ...try to get the message home to him ... but he just seems to shut off to it.   Father of Peter (age 15)

Anthony's father had come to a similar conclusion:

MR A: Well, I believe that this is all now, having been through the measures that we've been through - I believe this is all totally within his control (said calmly, but firmly)...Anthony - I suppose really as the result of the enuresis problem, has adopted the posture of not being a member of the family, in the social sense, he does things that he wants to do, he won't participate with the rest of us, he deliberately makes life difficult, now I believe that this is a conscious effort on his part to extract an attitude from the rest of us, so that he can heap more guilt on himself for the problem.

Father of Anthony (age 16)

In his search for meaning Anthony's father was suggesting that Anthony received some kind of benefit from "extracting an attitude" from the rest of the family. He also suggested that Anthony was using the bed wetting as an excuse for other areas in his life where he perceived himself as failing. A consultation with a urologist had only served to confirm this father's views:

> MR A: Eventually Mr B [the urologist] and I sat down with Anthony and we talked about it and I told Mr B that I felt that Anthony was quite capable of controlling the situation, that it has now reached the stage that it wasn't a physical problem, it was a psychological problem. And as soon as we arrived at the point at which Anthony wanted it to work, it would work. And I rather got the impression that Mr B had also arrived at the same point, because medically there was very little else that he could do.
>
> Father of Anthony (age 16)

Anthony's father's theory about the cause of his son's bed wetting was based on other evidence, as well:

> MR A: ... if he was serious about this, he would take the tablets. If he was serious in times gone past, about being dry, he would have filled the chart in, but it was always a question of 'Have you filled the chart in?' 'No'. So somebody else fills the chart in for him, whether it's good news or bad news. That doesn't say to me that he's actively involved in trying to want to resolve this problem.
>
> Father of Anthony (age 16)

The members of this family were locked in a self-perpetuating cycle of conflicting and strongly held beliefs, feelings and behaviour which had led to tension and distress for all concerned.

In contrast to the generally benevolent stance taken by Anthony's and Peter's fathers, the mother of Sarah (age 11) seemed to have taken a consistently punitive approach towards her daughter in situations both related and unrelated to bed wetting. Sarah's mother appeared to vacillate between pro-active rejection and intolerance and ambivalence towards her daughter's bed wetting. She said that she did at times feel very angry about it:

> MRS S: I mean I can sort of go off in a tirade and get really cross with her and tell her that I'm fed up with the smell ... and then you look at the child and you've got her feelings to consider, and then you feel sorry for what you've done, shouting and bawling. It's not her fault, you know, then you go on a guilt trip.
>
> Mother of Sarah (age 11)

The dilemma for Sarah's mother was whether or not her daughter could control the situation. This mother had wet the bed herself until she was 10 years old:

> MRS S: I can remember being in more control of it than I let on. I was lazy ... more often than not I was with Billy [her brother] so it could be Billy who did it, it didn't have to be me. She [her mother] never knew who it was ... I was just lazy. That is how I wonder if she's like that, if she's doing that - it is warm and cosy in bed, you don't want to get up to go to the toilet.
>
> Mother of Sarah (age 11)

Sarah's mother had punished her daughter in many ways for wetting the bed. She felt that health care professionals blamed her for her daughter's problems. She had tried and persisted with many treatments for her daughter's bed wetting but to no avail. She described her relationship with her daughter as poor and described her daughter as: "highly volatile", "manipulative", and "very secretive". The message sent to Sarah by her mother seems to be: "You could act differently and you are disobeying my wishes".

Before he had become reliably dry, through taking Triptizol, Martin's mother appeared to be sending her son the same message. When asked what his feelings had been when he did wet the bed, Martin replied:

> MARTIN: I cry ... 'You've to keep it dry'.
>
> Martin (age 6)

Martin's mother had insisted that he wear nappies and she had been intolerant of the bed wetting until she realised that her son could not help it.

Lazarus (1991) considers anger to be one of the most powerful emotions, which can have a profound impact on social relations as well as on the person experiencing the emotion. He suggests that what makes anger different from other negative emotional states (all of which he suggests derive from harm, loss or threats) is that blame is directed at someone or something.

To blame persons, rather than simply holding them accountable or responsible for harm, loss or threat suggests that the person believes that the object of their anger could have acted differently, that is they had control over the offending action. The inference is that the other person acted with volition, that is without proper regard for the sensibilities of the person offended.

Lazarus (1991) also suggests that any action that is deemed to be inconsiderate or malevolent contributes to the impression that the person has been demeaned, the angry person has suffered what is taken to be damage or threat to ego-identity, whether this is recognised consciously and admitted or not. He suggests that the word "offence" refers not merely to the frustration of a goal (though frustration certainly has emotional significance) but that it carries a special significance, namely a slight to the person's own self.

Lazarus suggests that a powerful impulse arising from anger is to exact vengeance, that is to attack the person held responsible for the offence. He suggests, however, that people may act benignly and constructively on the basis of threat, enlightened self-interest, or strongly internalised ethical values. In other words, a person's anger may not be translated directly into actions although it is unlikely that the anger will remain totally invisible.

Anger seemed to be a particularly common emotion amongst those parents whose attitude towards bed wetting is described as resigned reactive rejection and intolerance, as is described below.

Resigned reactive rejection and intolerance Resigned reactive rejection and intolerance is defined as rejection and intolerance of a situation which the parent believes is within the young person's control but outwith their (the parents') control. This attitude is described as resigned and reactive because the parent has given up trying to influence the situation and merely reacts to events as they occur, usually in a negative way.

All the parents exhibiting this attitude appeared to have, or to have had, a poor relationship with the young person more generally. These parents had also consistently and consciously punished their children for bed wetting. They were amongst the most angry as well as the most frustrated by it. In two cases the parents thought that the bed wetting was deliberate:

> MRS M: I mean she could get up but then there were nights she can be lazy. I mean you can walk into the room and she can be sitting up in the bed and says, 'I'm sorry, mum'. 'Right, OK'. And I just walk away.
>
> Mother of Michelle (age 8)

The relationship between Michelle and her mother did not appear to be good and her daughter was punished for other misdemeanours. Gary's father was similarly convinced that his son deliberately wet the bed. His wife described the relationship between Gary and his father as poor and she explained her perception of the situation:

> MRS G: I feel if Alan [her husband] has been shouting at him and annoying him, I think Gary deliberately wets the bed, because when he does wet the bed and his dad's shouting at him and that, Gary looks at his dad and you can see the hate in his eyes. Mother of Gary (age 5)

Gary's mother felt that this was a way in which Gary was able to retaliate when his father was angry with him because he knew that his father was unhappy about the bed wetting and particularly disliked the smell of the urine in the house.

Tracy's mother was also very angry about the bed wetting. She was finding it particularly difficult to manage four children on her own. Conversations within this household were chaotic experiences, in which arrangements to meet had been forgotten and the children could be found wandering through the house eating their meals at any time of the day. Perhaps for Tracy's mother the bed wetting was the last straw in a situation over which she already felt that she had very little control. Tracy's four year old sister had recently started wetting the bed as well and the girls shared a bedroom.

Life within the families of Michelle, Gary and Tracy seemed to be characterised by inter-personal conflict.

This group includes the three natural fathers who were said by their wives to have abdicated from all responsibility for helping the young person to learn to be dry at night or to manage the consequences arising from the bed wetting in the meantime.

These parents are sometimes scornful, contemptuous or disdainful of the young person's bed wetting. Ford (1992, p.150) describes the message attached to the emotion of "scorn - disdain - contempt" as:

You know better than that - shape up or ship out!

This is reminiscent of Stone's (1973) contention that bed wetting into adulthood can lead to rejection from the family and perhaps ultimately to homelessness, in some cases.

Certainly the nurturing quality displayed by accepting and tolerant parents in general, and by the ambivalent and proactive intolerant parents in situations other than bed wetting, seemed to be noticeably absent amongst those parents whose attitude was primarily one of resigned reactive rejection and intolerance. It is, however, not possible to say which came first - the poor relationship between the parent and the young person or the bed wetting.

It may be, in some cases, that the young person's behaviour in response to their parents' intolerance, makes them less easy to live with than other children within the same family. The situation may be one of "mutual simultaneous shaping" - a situation which is coming to be recognised in the family literature (e.g. Brodrick, 1993; Gelles, 1995; and Muncie et al, 1995).

Many of the intolerant parents were having to cope with other problems at the time of the study and could well have been experiencing a phenomenon referred to by Burr and Klein (1994) as "stress pile up".

Young people's beliefs about the causes of bed wetting

The beliefs of the young people in this study about the causes of their bed wetting are reviewed in this section and compared with the results of a recent survey. By themselves these beliefs do not seem to account for young people's differing attitudes towards their bed wetting and to treatment, or to account for their feelings about themselves as bed wetters.

The majority of the young people in this study had no idea what was causing their bed wetting, or why they were wetting the bed less often than before, when they were beginning to achieve some dry nights. Most felt that they had little or no control over the situation and expressed varying degrees of optimism about the future. Sarah's response was typical:

SARAH: I don't know why I do it, I just do it.   Sarah (age 11)

In an attempt to be helpful some young people cast about for a possible explanation. In innocence John put forward a theory suggested by a friend:

JOHN: Well my pal says, 'You must be having wet dreams'.   John (age 8)

In contrast to Butler's (1994) study, described below, Anthony was the only young person to suggest that his bed wetting could be due to deep sleep. Carol (age 17) thought that her bed wetting could be due to bad luck:

CAROL: It was my bad luck for breaking four mirrors ... 28 years bad luck! (laughs).

A little later on in the conversation, Carol offered a different explanation:

CAROL: It could be the mind ...
MOYA: In what sort of way?
CAROL: In what sort of way? Why did I come out with that idea! I dinnae know. It could be, that's all I'll say, it might be.
MOYA: Has anyone said that to you or is that your idea?
CAROL: Mine.   Carol (age 17)

It could be that other young people also had theories about the cause of their bed wetting, which they were reluctant to share. Perhaps they felt that their theory reflected badly on them as a person in some way. The inability of most of the younger children to articulate any explanation for their bed wetting may well be a reflection of the stage of their cognitive and linguistic development.

In a study by Butler (1994) fifty children were asked to rate each of eight statements about the possible "biological" cause of their bed wetting, using a 0 - 6 Likert Scale. "I sleep too deeply" (p. 18) received the highest mean rating . When presented with a schedule listing ten "psychological" causes these children rated: "Fail to wake to full bladder signals" and "Not learned to hold through the night" (p. 34 - 35) as the most likely causes of their bed wetting. These are all causes over which the young people perceived themselves to have little or no control.

Asking young people to rate predetermined options may give the rather misleading impression that they are more certain of the cause of their bed wetting than is actually the case. Most of the young people in the present study seemed genuinely perplexed about why they wet the bed. They were vague with their explanations which, for the most part, seemed to lack conviction.

It is argued below that young people's beliefs about their control over the bed wetting may be more potent determinants of both their attitudes and behaviour than the "biological" and "psychological" causes explored by Butler (1994).

Young people's attitudes towards bed wetting

As with parents, several factors have been found to transcend young people's specific attributional beliefs about bed wetting, as determinants of their overall attitude to it, their feelings about it and their responses to it. These include: their concern about the bed wetting; their desire to be dry; their belief in their capacity to influence the situation now and their optimism that they will one day be dry at night.

It is suggested that the young people's attitudes towards bed wetting can be classified into one of four broad categories: acceptance and tolerance; ambivalence; proactive rejection and intolerance, or resigned helplessness and hopelessness. The first category of acceptance and tolerance has been further subdivided according to the young people's concern about the bed wetting and optimism about becoming dry in the future. Table 5.3 therefore describes and summarises seven attitudes of young people towards bed wetting, together with some of their antecedents and consequences.

As with parents' attitudes, it is emphasised that these seven attitudes should not be regarded as consistent, stable traits. Rather, they are differing perspectives which young people bring to any situation they find themselves in relating to bed wetting. As with their parents, young people's perspectives may change over time.

Table 5.3
Young people's attitudes towards bed wetting

(The structure of this table is based on Strauss and Corbin's (1990) axial coding paradigm)   N/A = not applicable

	YOUNG PERSON'S ATTITUDE						
	ACCEPTANCE AND TOLERANCE				AMBIVALENCE	PROACTIVE REJECTION AND IN-TOLERANCE	RESIGNED HELPLESSNESS AND HOPELESSNESS
	Primary unconcerned	Happy	Resigned pragmatic	Optimistic pragmatic			
A. CAUSAL CONDITIONS							
1. The young person is concerned about the bed wetting	No	No	Yes	Yes	Yes/No	Yes	Yes
2. The young person believes that he/she has the capacity to control the situation now	NA	Yes, at least to some extent	No	Perhaps, to some extent	Perhaps, to some extent	Yes	No
3. The young person believes that he/she will one day be dry at night	NA	Yes	No	Yes	Not sure	Yes	Not sure

Table 5.3 continued

	YOUNG PERSON'S ATTITUDE						
	ACCEPTANCE AND TOLERANCE				AMBIVALENCE	PROACTIVE REJECTION AND IN-TOLERANCE	RESIGNED HELPLESSNESS AND HOPELESSNESS
	Primary unconcerned	Happy pragmatic	Resigned pragmatic	Optimistic pragmatic			
B. PHENOMENON The young person's overall attitude to the bed wetting	Young person accepts and tolerates a situation which he/she believes:				Young person has mixed feelings about a situation which he/she believes could perhaps be changed, but which may bring benefits, if at some personal cost	Young person does not accept and is no longer prepared to tolerate a situation that he/she believes can be changed now	Young person is resigned to a situation that he/she believes cannot be changed now and is unlikely to change
	is not a problem	brings benefits, if at some personal cost	is unlikely ever to change	could change soon			

C. INTERVENING CONDITIONS include:
1. Young person's belief in his/her competence in other tasks
2. Attitude of parents, siblings, wider family and friends towards the bed wetting
3. Attitude of health care professionals towards the bed wetting

Table 5.3 continued

	YOUNG PERSON'S ATTITUDE						
	ACCEPTANCE AND TOLERANCE				AMBIVA-LENCE	PROACTIVE REJECTION AND IN-TOLERANCE	RESIGNED HELPLESS-NESS AND HOPELESS-NESS
	Primary unconcerned	Happy	Resigned pragmatic	Optimistic pragmatic			
D. INTERACTIONAL STRATEGIES							
1. Accepts responsibility for learning to be dry at night, when treatments are available	NA	No	NA	Yes	Perhaps	Yes	Perhaps, but half-heartedly
2. Persists with treatment and regards failures as temporary setbacks	NA	No	NA	Yes	No	Yes, very persistent and determined	No, easily discouraged
E. CONSEQUENCES FOR YOUNG PERSON							
1. Feelings, in relation to bed wetting episodes	Unconcerned	Happy	Very sad	Sad, at times	Mixed feelings, sad at times	Angry, at him/her self	Very sad
2. Feelings of shame associated with the bed wetting more generally	No	No	Yes	Yes	Yes	Yes	Yes

It is suggested that young people may vacillate between two perspectives, for instance between optimistic pragmatism and resigned helplessness and hopelessness, in response to their evaluation of the success or otherwise of new initiatives to encourage the bed wetting to stop, which are usually undertaken at the parents' instigation. However, the attitudes of most young people appeared to have been consistently held for prolonged periods, in contrast to the attitudes of most parents which seemed more amenable to change. It is suggested that the difference in the stability of young people's and parents' attitudes is a reflection in part of the difference in the amount of control that young people and their parents perceive themselves to be able to exercise over their lives more generally and their differing access to strategies to help to overcome the situation.

Each of the attitudes summarised in Table 5.3 is described below, with illustrations from the young people's own accounts of their beliefs, feelings and behaviour, supported by secondary evidence from parents in some cases. Where terms such as "acceptance", "tolerance" and "rejection" have already been defined for parents, the same definitions are applied to the situations relating to the young people's attitudes.

Acceptance and tolerance

Four sub categories of acceptance and tolerance are summarised in Table 5.3.

Primary unconcerned acceptance and tolerance Primary unconcerned acceptance and tolerance is defined as acceptance and tolerance of a situation that the young person has not yet come to recognise as being a cause for concern. This attitude is described as primary because it is contended that young people do not begin life with feelings of shame about lack of bladder control but have to learn from others that wetting the bed is socially unacceptable behaviour. It is acknowledged that in very young children there is a stage which precedes this, when the child is not aware of "self" (Hetherington and Parke, 1993; Mussen et al, 1990).

Happy acceptance and tolerance Happy acceptance and tolerance is defined as acceptance and tolerance of a situation that the young person has discovered brings with it some secondary benefits, if at some personal cost. Butler (1987) suggests that deliberate bed wetting is rare. In the present study there was some evidence to suggest that Gary was wetting the bed deliberately and that Michelle had wet the bed deliberately on some occasions in the past.

The parents of both these children said that they had observed the child to

151

wet the bed while awake. Gary's mother had attributed her son's behaviour to his desire to retaliate when his father was angry with him over other issues. Gary was the only young person to indicate that he felt happy when he woke up to find the bed wet by ticking a smiling face on a faces-feelings card and he confirmed this in conversation alone with the researcher:

MOYA: Do you ever wet the bed?
GARY: Sometimes.
MOYA: Sometimes. And how do you feel about that?
GARY: Fine.
MOYA: You feel fine about it - you don't mind about it?
GARY: No.   Gary (age 5)

When asked if there were any bad things about wetting the bed, he replied: "getting skelped" (physically punished). Gary was consistently blamed by his father for bed wetting and was often punished for it. He did not, however, appear to be ashamed of the bed wetting. Gary was a secondary bed wetter.

The only other young person where there was the hint of happy acceptance of wetting the bed in the past was Michelle. Michelle appeared to have a poor relationship with her mother and she was often punished for bed wetting. At the time of the study Michelle said that she was sad about the bed wetting because of the smell and because she sometimes developed a rash. She ticked an unhappy face to describe how she felt when she found her bed wet:

MOYA: Tell me why that one.
MICHELLE: Because I want to get it over and done with.
MOYA: I'm sure.
MICHELLE: Because I don't like the bed wetting any more. Because when some people come to stay with me they'll find out.   Michelle (age 8)

Michelle's comments suggest that she had learned to be concerned about the bed wetting and wanted it to stop for social reasons. One of the greatest concerns of young people about their bed wetting was discovery by peers (Chapter 4).

Resigned pragmatic acceptance and tolerance Resigned pragmatic acceptance and tolerance is defined as acceptance and tolerance of a situation which the young person believes cannot be changed now and is highly unlikely to change ever. This attitude is described as pragmatic and resigned because the young person has realistically given up hope of becoming dry at night.

152

The young person is not blamed by his parents for behaviour which is recognised as being beyond his control but the young person nevertheless feels very sad and perhaps ashamed about his lack of ability to do what other young people can do. In this study there was only one young person who fell within this category, Michael, who had been diagnosed as having only one, partially functioning kidney shortly after birth. Michael was very sad about the bed wetting but in a rather different way from the other young people, as he explained when he described his picture of himself on a wet morning:

MOYA: And how do you feel?
MICHAEL: Sad about it. I actually feel kind of silly at times.
MOYA: Why is that?
MICHAEL: Because I think to myself - I can't do some of the things normal boys do. Michael (age 8)

To Michael, wetting the bed was an indication that he was different from other children.

Optimistic pragmatic acceptance and tolerance This attitude is defined as acceptance and tolerance of a situation which the young person believes could change soon. This attitude is described as optimistic and pragmatic because the young person believes that he is capable of achieving dry nights but is realistic that the achievement of this goal is unlikely to happen overnight or without effort.

For the most part these young people believe that their parents do not blame them or no longer blame them for wetting the bed but they do recognise that their parents are at times frustrated and angry about having to manage the consequences arising from the wet bed, especially the extra laundry.

At the time of this study nine young people seemed to have adopted this attitude. However in only two cases did it appear that this attitude had been consistently held over a prolonged period. Although neither boy liked waking up to a wet bed, William and Ian seemed to be the least concerned about the bed wetting. All the young people in this group were wetting the bed three nights per week or less at the time of their conversations with the researcher and could see from their own experience that dry nights were possible, even if these were not always perceived to be directly linked to their own efforts.

Outward acceptance of the situation should not be taken to mean that these young people do not feel sad and ashamed about the bed wetting on occasion, in response to the negative remarks of others, especially their peers:

ROGER: It hurts me sometimes ... You get used to it. Roger (age 14)

Anthony seemed to vacillate between optimistic pragmatism and resigned helplessness. During this study the frequency of his bed wetting fell quite markedly and he seemed optimistic and philosophical on speaking with the researcher after the diary keeping:

> ANTHONY: It's like sort of restrictive. I don't really class it as anything wrong, but it's just something I have to live with.   Anthony (age 16)

However Anthony's mother remarked that she had overheard her son talking to his younger sister Susan about his feelings:

> MRS A: Anthony's comment to Susan [his sister] was, 'a three-year old can do it and I can't. How'd you feel about that? How do you think I feel when a three or four year old child can be dry?' - and it was from the heart.
> Mother of Anthony (age 16)

Both Anthony and Roger had learned ways of coping with the bed wetting, at least outwardly. There was little doubt, however, that both of these young men were ashamed of bed wetting and that this had, at times, affected their self-esteem.

Some of the young people denied, at first, that they had much of a problem with their night time bladder control:

> JOHN: Before Christmas - I never wet until Christmas - well, last year I wet once because I was too excited. That was why I wet at Christmas. I was too excited.
> MOYA: Too excited. Any other times when it happens?
> JOHN: When it's my birthday.   John (age 8)

According to his urinary symptom questionnaire and diary John was actually wetting the bed 2-3 nights a week.

As discussed, for instance, by Lazarus (1991) and by Weiner (1992), it is commonplace for people who perceive themselves to have failed to achieve a personal ideal to desire to avoid having this failure observed by others. Feelings of shame lead to attempts to hide the failing from public exposure as the expectation is that others will disapprove, leading to a further lowering of their self-esteem.

Ambivalence

This attitude is defined as having mixed feelings about a situation which the young person believes could perhaps be changed but which he or she has discovered brings with it some benefits, if at some personal cost.

It was difficult to be sure what Sarah and Tracy felt about their bed wetting. Both seemed to be ambivalent about it. Both found it difficult to talk about their feelings. When asked to draw a picture of themselves on waking up in the morning to find themselves wet, both at first drew a happy face and then changed it. When asked who the smiling face belonged to Tracy replied:

> TRACY: That was me, but I did it wrong ... I meant to do it sad, but I done it happy. Tracy (age 9)

Sarah also altered her picture of herself on a wet morning before giving it to the researcher. Her mother pounced on this "mistake" immediately and said it was "highly significant". She said that she felt that Sarah had far more control over the situation than she "let on".

Whether or not Sarah or Tracy received any secondary benefits from wetting the bed, in terms of extra attention or were merely reluctant on some occasions to get out of a warm bed to go to the toilet is not known, but both girls appeared to be unhappy and both mothers described their relationships with their daughters as problematic. Tracy's mother described her daughter as "deep":

> MRS T: She kind of keeps things in, ken, she'll no' communicate, ken - she'll just no' sit and talk to you. Mother of Tracy (age 9)

Both Sarah and Tracy were living in households where conflict with their parents was common, and where they were consistently blamed and punished for their failure to fulfil their parents' expectations of them. Both parents seemed to be saying to their daughters that they could act differently if they chose to.

Proactive rejection and intolerance

This attitude is defined as a refusal to accept and endure a situation which the young person believes is within his control, given sufficient effort. The attitude is described as proactive because the young person accepts responsibility for the situation, persisting with treatment and perhaps even taking the initiative when new opportunities arise to enable the bed wetting to stop. The young person is determined to resolve the problem and is angry with himself for the continuance of a situation which it is believed could by now have been resolved with more effort. The continuance of the problem

155

leads to a reduction in the young person's self-esteem, which may in these cases, be a potent driving force for seeking a solution.

Two young people seemed to have adopted this attitude, Simon and Paul. Both appeared to be acutely embarrassed about the bed wetting and to want it to stop. The parents of both Simon and Paul were very supportive of their sons' efforts to be dry.

Simon had been making a consistent effort to be dry at night for some time before the study and he achieved two weeks of dry nights between completing the urinary symptom questionnaire and the first (and only) visit by the researcher, in spite of the fact that he had stopped taking Desmospray. In his picture of himself on waking up to find the bed wet he included his star chart on which he had faithfully marked his progress towards his goal of becoming dry. The inclusion of the star chart was unsolicited. When asked what his picture meant, he replied:

SIMON: I'm annoyed I'm wet.   Simon (age 8)

Simon seemed particularly determined to be dry and his mother was both optimistic, pragmatic and supportive. She said that she did not believe in punishment and she had discovered that even the use of small rewards had put too much pressure on Simon to be dry at times. She had discontinued using a rigid system of rewards which Simon had been unable to attain.

Paul was one of the most reluctant young people to speak with the researcher and appeared to be acutely embarrassed about the situation. Although he had agreed to the meeting when his parents had discussed this with him, he took the long way home from school on the day that the meeting was scheduled and hid behind the door of the room where the meeting was taking place.

Paul's father had encouraged him to take responsibility for the situation. He described his son as "fed up" with the bed wetting. Before the study Paul had taken responsibility for an alarm clock method which seemed to have worked well for him. This method had been suggested by a hypnotherapist.

Paul did not keep the study diary, but according to his father's Filofax he only wet the bed on 3 out of the 28 nights following the first meeting with the researcher. In each case there was said by his father to be mitigating circumstances. The researcher was left with the impression that Paul was angry that he had been involved in the study. According to the urinary symptom questionnaire he had been wetting the bed three nights a week on average but this had reduced to less than once a week during the time when the diary would have been kept. It was discovered eight months later, when his mother wrote to the researcher that Paul had become reliably dry shortly after his first meeting with the researcher, much to the delight of everyone in the family. This could have happened purely by chance, as 15 per cent of young people become spontaneously dry every year. Paul clearly wanted the bed wetting to stop and had accepted responsibility for helping it to stop. This may have contributed to his ultimate success.

Resigned helplessness and hopelessness

This attitude is defined as accepting with sadness a situation which the young person believes is outwith his or her control and is unlikely to change.

Unlike resigned pragmatism, the young person believes himself to be responsible and to be held responsible by one or both parents for a situation which he believes himself to be unable to influence, in the light of repeated failure to achieve dry nights, however hard he has tried in the past.

If these young people do engage in treatment suggested by others, their efforts are at best half-hearted and they are easily discouraged and give up quickly in the face of failure. They come to believe that any dry nights that they do experience are due to chance and they are ashamed that they cannot achieve an "easy" task, which most three year olds can accomplish. Their lack of belief in their ability to influence the situation and their lack of action is often interpreted by parents as a lack of concern about the bed wetting accompanied by a lack of effort to help themselves. They therefore perceive themselves to be, and are sometimes, blamed for doing too little to help themselves and they may have been punished in the past for their failure to comply with the behaviour expected by others.

In all, four young people were deemed to have this attitude at the time of the study. For a further three young people this seemed to have been their predominant attitude towards the bed wetting until the time of the study when they experienced that dry nights were possible. All seven of these young people had been wetting the bed on six to seven nights per week. All of these young people had also had problems with day wetting. This group included the four young people who had a day wetting problem "very often", with the urine usually leaking to the outside of their clothes. Six of the seven had had a day wetting episode at school and in four cases this had been recent. This group therefore included some of the most severely affected bed wetters, most of whom had had to live with the double disadvantage of lack of day time bladder control.

Carol was sad and frustrated about the bed wetting and clearly wanted it to stop. She was, however, pessimistic about the future:

MOYA: When do you think you're going to be dry? Have you got any ideas?

CAROL: No.

MOYA: No idea when it's going to happen?

CAROL: I'll just have to wait.

MOYA: You said when I spoke to you last, 'if I ever become dry', do you think you will become dry?

CAROL: Hopefully, yes. But doubtfully, no.   Carol (age 17)

Carol had tried many treatments but none had been successful. There was evidence to suggest that her attempts to become dry, at least latterly, had been at best half-hearted. Carol had suggested that the bed wetting might be due to bad luck or to something "in the mind". Carol's mother had wet the bed herself until she was 16 years of age and her father had wet the bed until he was 24 years old. This could well have affected Carol's expectancy that dry nights were possible.

Peter and Shelly also each had a parent who had not been dry until the age of 15 years. Peter had come to believe that he was unable to be dry, he therefore expected failure and he felt ashamed at his lack of ability to do what his 2½ year old half brother could do.

Shelly, like Peter, was very sad about the bed wetting and wanted it to stop. Although Shelly was wetting the bed every night of the week, according to her urinary symptom questionnaire, and the first three weeks of her diary, her parents had bought her a new bed at the time that they bought new beds for everyone else in the family and, as the diary records, Shelly then had six dry nights in a row. Her mother seemed genuinely astonished:

MRS S: I just couldn't believe it when she stopped wetting ... she's been great.   Mother of Shelly (age 7)

The bed had not been purchased with the intention of motivating Shelly to be dry or with any expectation that dry nights would result. However, Shelly may have taken the purchase of the new bed to be an indication that her mother thought that she was capable of achieving dry nights. She beamed with pleasure as she shyly told the researcher how many dry nights she had achieved in the week before the researcher's return visit.

At the start of this study Alison was obviously both sad and ashamed about wetting the bed. She had wet the bed almost every night for the previous seven years. Her mother had given up hope that she would ever be dry and had finally taken the conscious decision to do nothing more as everything that she had tried had failed. However Alison meticulously kept the study diary, under her mother's supervision and with both parents' encouragement, and she began to experience more and more dry nights. Through the diaries Alison came to see that she could be dry. She began to feel more in control of the situation and her feelings became much more positive as did the feelings of the whole family. This was reflected in the mother's diary. The entries for three mornings are given below:

> *Saturday, 26 March*: Alison a bit teary this morning and a bit upset with J [her stepfather]. Not a good day for her but at least she does try.
> *Wednesday, 30 March*: We're all very pleased that Alison is dry this morning. It just sets the day up the right way for us all.
> *Wednesday, 6 April*: Alison is dry again. This is the 6th morning she has been dry and over the moon. Her chart has gave her a lot of confadense [sic].   Extract from Alison's mother's diary, kept during the study

These extracts show the effects of bed wetting or a dry bed on the young person's feelings and behaviour in the morning, and the difference in the atmosphere within the household when the young person is dry. This is a clear illustration of mutual simultaneous shaping. Alison's mother commented on the difference in her daughter's behaviour in the mornings:

> MRS A: If she's dry now she'll come through running, 'I'm dry this morning!' - fairly proud of herself. When she's wet, she'll no' mention it - sometimes she'll say, 'I don't know', and she'll go back and checks and comes back. If she says 'I don't know', it usually means 'aye', when she tries to hide it.   Mother of Alison (age 9)

The above quotation illustrates the young person's pride in her achievement when dry, which she attributed to her own efforts and her feelings of shame when she could not live up to her own ideal, which she tried to hide.

In summary, most young people are sad and ashamed about wetting the bed and want it to stop but they vary widely in their belief in their own capacity to influence the situation and in their optimism about what the future holds.

The social origins of parents' and young people's beliefs and attitudes towards bed wetting

Social psychologists suggest that people are not born with beliefs and attitudes, although they may be born with a genetic predisposition towards them (Baron and Byrne, 1994). Rather it is thought that beliefs and attitudes are gradually acquired or learned, for the most part, from authoritative figures such as parents and teachers. This is sometimes referred to as social learning:

> Children learn from parents not only what objects *are* but what one should *believe* and *feel* about them and how one should *act* toward them
>
> Bernstein et al (1991) p.687

Social learning occurs in several ways, which include: classical conditioning; instrumental conditioning and modelling (Baron and Byrne, 1994; Stahlberg and Frey, 1994; Stroebe and Jonas, 1994). Learning can occur even when parents have no desire to transmit specific views to their children who, nevertheless, learn through observing their parents' behaviour. Children may carry many of their attitudes with them into parenthood. Beliefs and attitudes are also acquired from direct personal experience. Research suggests that attitudes learned in this way are more confidently and consistently held and are more resistant to change than attitudes borrowed from others (Baron and Byrne, 1994).

The social origins of parents' beliefs and attitudes towards bed wetting

It is not possible to know the myriad situations and experiences which have contributed to a person's beliefs and attitudes, however some of the possible sources of parents' beliefs and attitudes towards bed wetting are suggested in Figure 5.7. These sources are briefly commented upon below.

Prevailing social-cultural beliefs and the beliefs and attitudes of wider family and friends Irrespective of their own beliefs and attitudes towards their child's bed wetting, all the parents in this study believed that there were many people outwith the family, living in the local community and the wider society, who disapproved of bed wetting in children over a certain age. In many cases this belief was born of or confirmed by experience, when their child's bed wetting was discovered by others (Chapter 4).

Parents gave the disapproval of others as the main reason for their unease about letting the young person stay away from home. In practice some of the parents' close relatives were accepting of the situation and were happy to have the young person to stay but many were not. Fear of discovery was acknowledged by many parents, as well as by the young people themselves.

In his book: *Adult bed wetters and their problems,* Stone (1973, p.1) wrote:

> Even in these 'enlightened' times, it is commonly assumed that the complaint is somehow recriminatory on the sufferer.

160

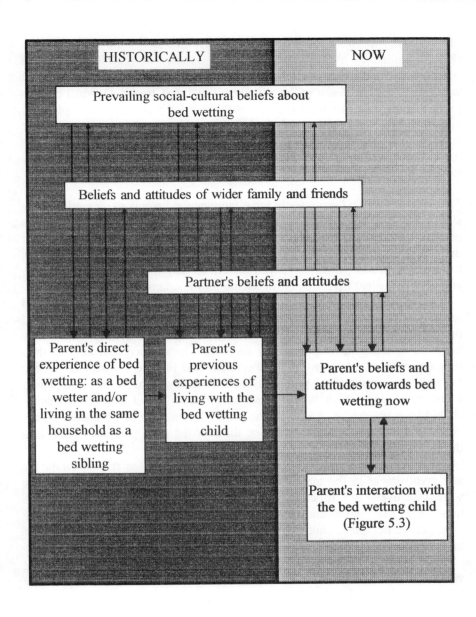

**Figure 5.7   Some possible sources of a parent's
beliefs and attitudes towards bed wetting**

In spite of the work of the Enuresis Resource and Information Centre (ERIC), initiatives of the Association for Continence Advice (ACA) and others, lack of bladder control can lead to feelings of shame in people of whatever age in response to the attitudes of others (Chapter 1). Most parents in this study did not perceive the attitude of others to be accepting or empathetic towards their child's bed wetting. There was some evidence to suggest that parents' attitudes were similar to their own parents' attitudes towards bed wetting, that is there seemed to be an intergenerational tendency towards either acceptance or intolerance of it.

Partners' beliefs and attitudes In most families the parents expressed broadly similar views about the young person's bed wetting, although many mothers commented that their husbands tended to be or to have been less tolerant of it than they were themselves. Parents described differences in their attitudes towards the use of punishment, with fathers tending towards a more punitive approach. This had been a cause of tension in some families.

There is some evidence that a mother's attitude towards her child's bed wetting is influenced by her perception of herself in the role of "mother" and the expectancy of others of her in this role (Chapter 4). Some mothers may have persuaded their husbands into adopting a more accepting attitude than they naturally felt. In many cases the father had little to do with the young person's bed wetting in the practical sense and many of these fathers appeared to be deferring to their wives' views and wishes about how the situation should be managed. In this sense the mother seemed to be orchestrating the views of both parents in the family so that, for the most part, they both sang the same tune.

In three cases, however, the father had clearly abdicated responsibility for any involvement in the management of the bed wetting and these mothers were effectively left to cope alone. These fathers were sending a clear message to their wives and children that the bed wetting was unacceptable. Whether or not these mothers felt blamed for the young person's lack of bladder control is not known.

In two families the mothers expressed mixed feelings about their sons' bed wetting in the light of their husbands' assertion that these adolescents had more control over the situation than they were choosing to exercise. Fathers may have more influence over the social environment created within the home for the young person to learn to be dry at night than has hitherto been realised. When assessing families it would seem prudent not to ignore the fathers' views.

Experience of being a bed wetter or living with a bed wetting sibling
A parent's experience of being a bed wetter or of living with a bed wetting sibling seemed to have a powerful influence on the parents' attitudes and beliefs about their own child's bed wetting. Mothers who had been bed wetters seemed to be particularly accepting of the young person's bed wetting while some fathers who had been bed wetters were clearly not (Chapter 4).

When discussing the methods that they had adopted to encourage the young person's bed wetting to stop several of the mothers who had themselves been bed wetters commented that they were only doing with their children what their mothers had done with them:

> MRS J: We had the buzzer. She [her mother] used to lift and lay us too. We weren't allowed drinks. It's only doing like what my mum did with us, really. Mother of John and Stephen (age 8)

The decision of mothers not to punish their child for bed wetting was also said to be a reflection of their own experience in some cases. These mothers did not punish their children either because they had not been punished themselves or because they had seen from their own experience that punishment did not hasten the achievement of dry beds.

Mothers who had personal experience of bed wetting were among the most optimistic that the young person would one day be dry, because they knew from their own experience that they themselves had become dry and they were among the most accepting and pragmatic of all parents in the meantime. There was, however, the suggestion that at least one mother had made very little effort on her child's behalf because she did not regard the bed wetting as a problem. It may also be that she did not regard bed wetting as particularly amenable to treatment, as a result of her own experiences as a bed wetter until the age of 15 when the bed wetting was said to have spontaneously resolved.

Previous experience with this young person A parent's previous experience of the bed wetting of their own child, discussed throughout Chapters 4 and 5, appeared to be a particularly important determinant of their expectancy of a successful outcome and of their feelings of control. The parents of seven young people who were wetting the bed six to seven nights per week, and for whom many treatments had failed, were among the most pessimistic about the outcome in the longer term and about their own ability to influence the situation, and understandably so.

Predispositional tendencies towards certain attitudes There is a small but growing body of evidence to suggest that genetic factors can play a part in attitude formation (Baron and Byrne, 1994; Plomin, 1994). Individuals may be born with a tendency towards optimism or pessimism, tolerance or intolerance, and feelings of competence or helplessness. A discussion of the influence of a parent's personal traits on his or her evaluation and interpretation of events is only touched upon, yet it could be an important contributory factor.

The social origins of young people's beliefs about bed wetting and about themselves as bed wetters

In this section it is argued that young people acquire their beliefs and attitudes towards bed wetting through a process of social learning, in much the same way that their parents have learned their beliefs and attitudes towards it. Young people learn to feel ashamed of wetting the bed as a result of the negative evaluation of their behaviour by others, both within and outwith the family. As a result of repeated failure to accomplish a task believed to be within the capability of a three year old, the young person's feelings of embarrassment and shame are reinforced and many young people come to believe that the outcome is not contingent upon their efforts. Young people may be born with a predisposition towards optimism or pessimism and with a belief in their own competence or helplessness to influence situations.

Learning to feel ashamed about wetting the bed It is suggested that young people learn to feel ashamed of wetting the bed as a result of the negative evaluation of their behaviour by others, both within and outwith the family. Lazarus (1991, p.241) describes the antecedents of shame:

> Shame is generated by a *failure to live up to an ego-ideal*. We feel disgraced or humiliated, especially in the eyes of someone whose opinion is of great importance to us such as a parent or parent-substitute [e.g. teacher, health care professional, perhaps] ... In shame, another person whose approbation is important to us views and presumably is critical of our failure. We have, in effect, disappointed that person ...

Weiner (1992) suggests that shame involves negative self evaluation and results from an internal ascription for some negative act or failure, leading to lowered self esteem.

Many parents described their children as embarrassed and ashamed about their bed wetting and most young people were fearful of the social consequences should their bed wetting be discovered by others. Even the most accepting parents gave fear of the disapproval of others as the principal reason for their unease about letting the young person stay away from home. It is suggested that these parents had sent the message to the young person: "We understand that you cannot help wetting the bed but there are people outwith the household who might disapprove. We don't want you to be hurt by the negative attitude of others". The young person does not need to experience disapproval directly to learn that bed wetting is regarded by some people as unacceptable behaviour after a certain age, however the data suggest that most young people had also had direct experience of the disapproval of others, including wider family and friends and had in some cases been publicly humiliated (Chapter 4).

In some cases the source of disapproval was other family members. Often the siblings' evaluation was perceived by the young person to be negative, especially if the sibling shared a bedroom with the bed wetter. It is suggested, however, that it is the parents' attitude towards the bed wetting, whether this is acceptance and tolerance, ambivalence or rejection and intolerance which is a particularly important determinant of the young person's attitudes towards bed wetting and towards himself as a bed wetter. Parents' disapproval was most clearly demonstrated by the consistent use of punishment for bed wetting.

An observation made in this study was that families varied in the consistency with which the young person's bed wetting was negatively evaluated by members of the same household, as is illustrated in Figure 5.8.

It was noticed that in one family the consensus with which the young person's bed wetting was negatively evaluated was high (Figure 5.8, pattern 1). Both Sarah's parents were intolerant of the bed wetting and her father had abdicated all responsibility for helping his daughter and his wife with it. Sarah's older sister was also said to be disapproving:

MRS S: ... my husband is not the least bit interested in it and her sister [age 16] thinks it's dirty and smelly and doesn't want to know.

Mother of Sarah (age 11)

Sarah's grandmother would not let her granddaughter stay in her house or caravan. Sarah herself seemed to be ambivalent in her attitude to the bed wetting.

In two families, the families of Peter (age 15) and Anthony (age 16), the father was intolerant of the bed wetting and the mother was ambivalent about it. Anthony's sister Susan (age 15) disapproved of it as well (Figure 5.8, pattern IIA). Anthony and Peter seemed to vacillate between optimistic pragmatism and resigned helplessness and hopelessness, but for the most part tended towards the latter perspective.

165

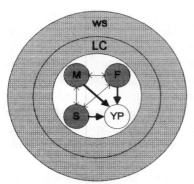

I High consensus towards
negative evaluation

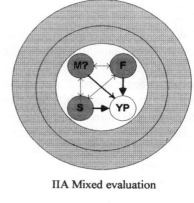

IIA Mixed evaluation

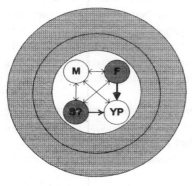

IIB Mixed evaluation

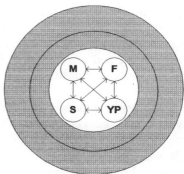

III Low consensus, with bed
wetting accepted within the
family home

<u>KEY</u> (see also Figure 3.1)

<u>OUTWITH THE FAMILY SYSTEM</u>
(= SUPRASYSTEM)

WS = wider society
LC = members of the local community e.g.
extended family, friends and neighbours.

 = regard bed wetting as inappropriate
for the young person's age
(individuals may or may not be
intolerant of the bed wetting)

<u>WITHIN THE FAMILY SYSTEM</u>
M = mother F = father S = sibling
YP = young person who wets the bed
Individual member's attitudes to the
bed wetting:

 = rejection and intolerance

 = ambivalence

 = acceptance and tolerance

**Figure 5.8   The consistency with which the young person's bed wetting
is negatively evaluated by others, within and outwith the
family**

166

In three families one of the parents was intolerant of the bed wetting but one was not (Figure 5.8, pattern IIB). In Gary's family the father was intolerant of the bed wetting but the mother was not. Gary (age 5) seemed happy about wetting the bed, for the most part. In Michelle's family, the mother was more intolerant of the situation than her second husband, who seemed to accept it but had little practical involvement with it. By the time of the study Michelle (age 8) seemed anxious that the bed wetting should stop but there was evidence to suggest that she may have been happy about it when she was younger. Tracy's mother was also intolerant of her daughter's bed wetting. By the time of the study Tracy's natural father, who had had little involvement in the management of bed wetting, had left the family home. Tracy seemed to be ambivalent in her attitude towards the bed wetting.

At the time of the study the parents in 13 of the 19 families seemed to have adopted an attitude of acceptance and tolerance and there was little evidence that the siblings were consistently disapproving (Figure 5.8, pattern III). The attitude of the young people in these families varied widely from resigned or optimistic pragmatic acceptance, to rejection and intolerance or resigned helplessness and hopelessness. However, in only three families did it appear that an attitude of optimistic pragmatism had been consistently held by the parents and in each case the young person was optimistic about the future and only minimally concerned about the bed wetting in the mean time. The young people in these families were, nevertheless, aware of the negative evaluation of bed wetting by people outwith the family and two of the three had learned to be fearful of the consequences of their bed wetting being discovered by others.

The consequences of the emotion of shame Attribution theorists, such as Weiner (1992), suggest that shame results when failure is attributed to lack of ability. Weiner (1992) and Lazarus (1991) suggest that as a consequence of experiencing shame the individual experiences further loss of control, feels powerless and usually withdraws from public contact. As Lazarus (1991, p.244) describes it, the action tendency accompanying shame is:

> ... to hide, to avoid having one's personal failure observed by anyone, especially someone who is personally important. To publicly expose one's failure to live up to an ego-ideal is to risk disapproval and quite possibly even rejection.

Young people's feelings of shame about wetting the bed were suggested in so many ways including: their humiliation on being put back into nappies; their hiding of wet night-clothes and their reluctance to tell their parents in the morning that the bed was wet; their avoidance of staying away with friends, in some cases; their reluctance to discuss their bed wetting with friends; their reluctance to admit that siblings and friends knew about the problem, and their non-verbal behaviour when discussing the bed wetting with the researcher.

In this study children as young as four years of age had learned to feel ashamed of wetting the bed. Only one young person did not seem fully aware that his bed wetting behaviour might be disapproved of by others. In this case the mother had gone to great lengths to protect her son from the disapproval of others.

Many parents commented on the difference in the young person's behaviour on "dry" mornings, when the young person was reported to be much more sociable. One mother also commented upon the difference in her son's behaviour at bed times once he had become dry.

It is suggested that the consequences of the negative emotion of shame for the young person's motivation to be dry is usually motivational inhibition (Weiner, 1992) but if the young person comes to believe that some control might be possible then shame can lead to a redoubling of efforts, as illustrated by the cases of Simon and Paul in this study.

The consequences of the disapproval of others for the young person's self concept more generally are now described.

The effect of bed wetting on self concept Self concept is defined by Burns (1980, p.171) as the set of attitudes a person holds towards himself. Burns suggests that self concept is composed of two elements: self image and self esteem. Self image is a self-picture, the answer to the question, "Who am I?" which contains all the person's perceived attributes, self conceptualisations, role and status characteristics, possessions and goals. Self esteem is defined by Burns (1980, p.174) as the evaluation or judgement placed on each element of the self image. Self esteem is therefore multi-dimensional. Mussen et al (1990) suggest that although children seem to have a general sense of self worth, self esteem varies for different domains of behaviour.

In the present study most of the young people seemed to have a positive view of themselves in general although they were, for the most part, unhappy about and ashamed of their bed wetting and wanted it to stop. This is congruent with the findings of Butler (1994), Moffatt et al (1987), and Wagner and Geffken (1986), who found that the children in their study had a relatively positive view of themselves, which they assessed using their Child Attitude Scale (CAS).

In the present study no formal instruments were used to measure the young person's self esteem. Measuring self esteem in children is fraught with methodological difficulties. According to Mussen et al (1990, p.391) pre-school children almost always say that they are satisfied and happy with themselves, "accompanying their comments with a slightly mystified look". Mussen et al (1990) suggest that children have a more clearly formulated sense of self worth and competence by the age of nine or ten but from this age they may not want to admit to others that they have undesirable qualities and they may report more positive self esteem than they really feel.

Many factors are known to affect a young person's feelings of self worth including family disruption and breakdown (Amato, 1986a,b; Burghes, 1994; Cockett and Tripp, 1994; Hetherington, 1989; Mennen and Meadow, 1994), parents' behaviour towards the young person more generally (Clarke-Stewart, 1988; Gecas and Schwalbe, 1986; Lamborn et al, 1991) and the appraisal of the young person by teachers at school (Graham, 1990). All that can be said is that negative self evaluation as a result of wetting the bed may contribute to the young person's overall sense of self worth which is derived from many sources. If the young person has developed a negative self image from other sources, negative self evaluation as a result of bed wetting may add to this. If the young person has a more positive self image on the whole, it may be easier for him or her to accept that lack of bladder control is an isolated instance of lack of competence.

The reinforcement of parents' and young people's attitudes as family members interact from day to day

Seen from a systems perspective and the naturalist paradigm, which emphasise mutual simultaneous shaping, the concept of linear causality is illogical. The emphasis shifts from seeing parents' actions as the "cause" of outcomes for the child (a psychological approach to the family and child development which dominated family research from the 1950s to the 1970s) to an attempt to understand the influence that family members exert on each other, through their words and actions. Communication is seen as a jointly constructed activity in which participants mutually evoke verbal and non-verbal messages and modify their own messages in response to the feedback that they receive.

The section begins by describing the origins of the conceptual model which illustrates the relationship between beliefs, feelings and behaviour as a parent and a young person interact from day to day. It is shown that the inferences drawn by young people and their parents as they seek to interpret each others' behaviour tend to reinforce their own personally held beliefs, which may be tenaciously held, even in the presence of conflicting evidence. It is argued that the social and emotional environment created for the young person to learn the skill of becoming dry at night is a reflection of the attitudes that each party brings to it and acts out. It is suggested that the nature of the young person's response also affects the nature of the parent's experience of bed wetting.

The origins of the conceptual model

The conceptual model illustrated at Figure 5.3 (p.119) had as its origins a logic diagram drawn by the researcher in an attempt to determine the sequence of events as a young person and his parents interpreted and responded to each other's behaviour on a "wet" morning (Figure 5.9).

This figure is based on an analysis of a single case, that of Peter (age 15) and his parents. The "event" is described more fully by Peter's step father:

> MR P: ... he gets up in the morning and he is - he has a shower. He spends maybe 20 minutes in the shower as if he wants to purify himself and get rid of everything a million per cent, so he walks out as a clean person and just leaves the bed behind for somebody else to deal with.
>
> MOYA: And how do you feel about that?
>
> MR P: I don't know - I think to a certain extent its a psychological problem with Peter - that he just seems to shut off - he doesn't want to face up to the problem.   Father of Peter (age 15)

This story has many features in common with other parents' descriptions of their children's behaviour on "wet" mornings (Chapter 4).

The inferences that Peter's parents had drawn from their son's behaviour were that he was not concerned about the bed wetting or was not prepared to face up to it, he was not making sufficient effort to help himself and he was not playing his part as a member of the family. At times, his parents felt angry, frustrated and helpless. On one occasion Peter's father videoed his stepson's response to being woken up in the night, to let him see what he was like, to which Peter was said to have replied:

> MR P: [quoting Peter]... 'I wet the bed - I believe you, you've proved your point!'   Father of Peter (age 15)

Peter's father had hoped that making his son face the problem would shock him into doing something about it. It was not, however, said to have made any difference to Peter's behaviour. There was no evidence that Peter's parents had used physical punishment although they had come to believe that the bed wetting was, to some extent, within his control.

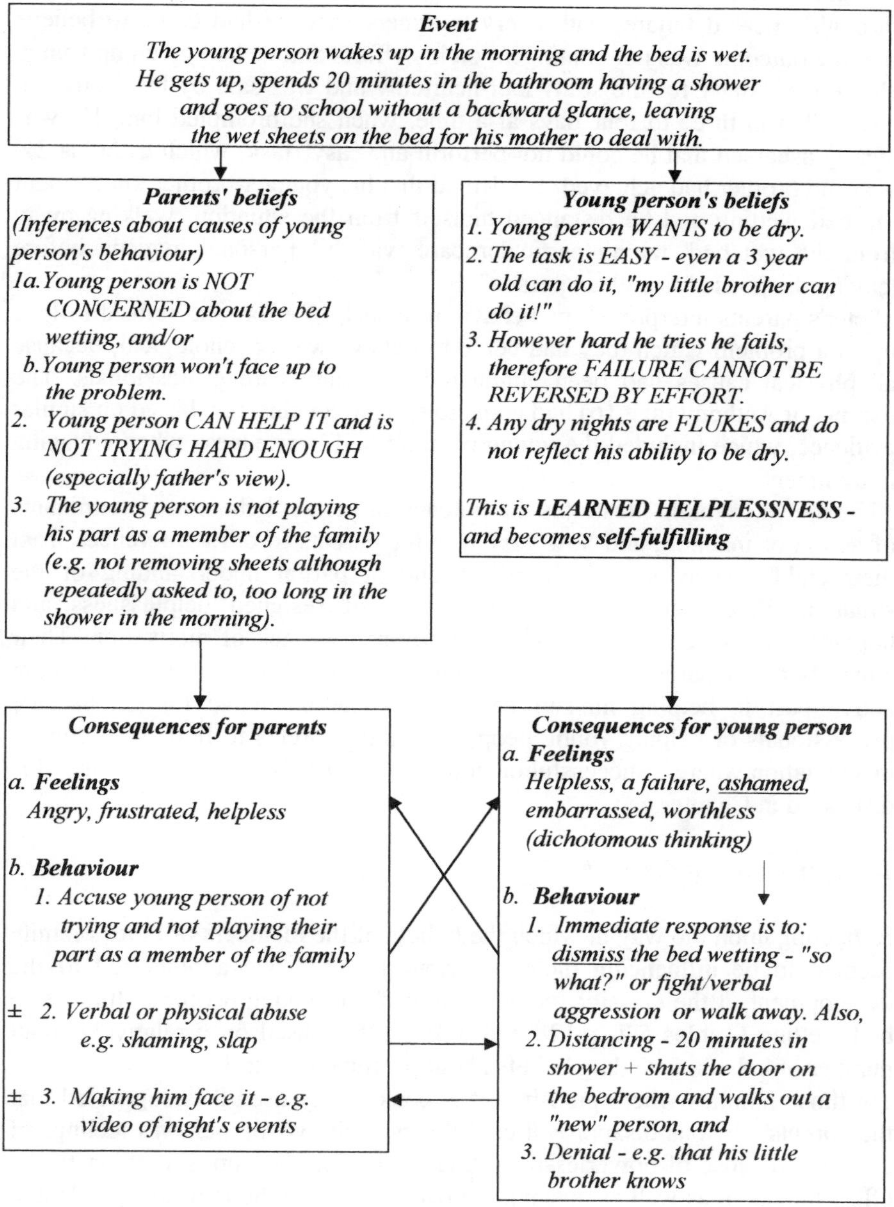

Event
The young person wakes up in the morning and the bed is wet.
He gets up, spends 20 minutes in the bathroom having a shower
and goes to school without a backward glance, leaving
the wet sheets on the bed for his mother to deal with.

Parents' beliefs
(Inferences about causes of young person's behaviour)
1a. Young person is NOT CONCERNED about the bed wetting, and/or
 b. Young person won't face up to the problem.
2. Young person CAN HELP IT and is NOT TRYING HARD ENOUGH (especially father's view).
3. The young person is not playing his part as a member of the family (e.g. not removing sheets although repeatedly asked to, too long in the shower in the morning).

Young person's beliefs
1. Young person WANTS to be dry.
2. The task is EASY - even a 3 year old can do it, "my little brother can do it!"
3. However hard he tries he fails, therefore FAILURE CANNOT BE REVERSED BY EFFORT.
4. Any dry nights are FLUKES and do not reflect his ability to be dry.

This is **LEARNED HELPLESSNESS** - and becomes *self-fulfilling*

Consequences for parents

a. *Feelings*
 Angry, frustrated, helpless

b. *Behaviour*
 1. Accuse young person of not trying and not playing their part as a member of the family

± 2. Verbal or physical abuse e.g. shaming, slap

± 3. Making him face it - e.g. video of night's events

Consequences for young person
a. *Feelings*
 Helpless, a failure, <u>ashamed</u>, embarrassed, worthless (dichotomous thinking)

b. *Behaviour*
 1. Immediate response is to: <u>dismiss</u> the bed wetting - "so what?" or fight/verbal aggression or walk away. Also,
 2. Distancing - 20 minutes in shower + shuts the door on the bedroom and walks out a "new" person, and
 3. Denial - e.g. that his little brother knows

Figure 5.9 An example of a logic diagram: "*What is going on?*"

Peter's beliefs are also summarised in Figure 5.9. Peter wanted to be dry but through repeated failure, with every treatment tried he had come to believe that the outcome was not contingent on his efforts and he had given up trying. He kept his diary for the study half-heartedly and was said by his mother to have filled in three to four days at a time, when she prompted him. He was clearly ashamed that he could not perform an "easy" task, which even his 2½ year old brother had achieved. He denied that his younger brother knew about the bed wetting and he distanced himself from the situation, walking away from the wet bed, taking particular care with his personal hygiene before leaving the house "as a clean person".

Peter's parents interpreted his behaviour as lack of effort and refusal to face up to a problem which they had come to believe was psychological, because all physical causes had been eliminated by health care professionals. The parents of Anthony (age 16) had come to similar conclusions, based on similar evidence, which included the young person's half-heartedness when engaging in treatment.

The above example illustrates the potency of certain beliefs as determinants of action or inaction, and how easy it is for parents to draw inferences from their child's behaviour which reflect only a partial understanding of the situation. Peter had come to an attitude of resigned helplessness and hopelessness which his parents had interpreted as lack of motivation. Their attempts to encourage him to take more responsibility and to play a more active part in helping himself had failed. The challenge for health care professionals of helping young people and their parents to find some control in a situation where a successful outcome to treatment cannot be guaranteed is discussed in Chapter 6.

The application of the model

Reflecting upon the way in which the beliefs of the members of Peter's family seemed to be influencing their behaviour towards one another led to the development of the classifications of parents' and young people's attitudes to bed wetting (Tables 5.2, p.128 and 5.3, p.148), based on a relatively small number of beliefs, including beliefs about perceived control.

In those families where punishment is consistently used it is suggested that the parents' obvious disapproval contributes to the young person's feelings of shame and sense of powerlessness, thereby having the opposite effect to the effect intended, as well as pushing the bed wetting up the family's agenda and increasing tension between family members at key times of communal family activity. Tracy's mother described what happened on the mornings when she found her daughter's bed was wet:

MRS T: I just shout at her - I do shout. I say 'Wet again!' you ken. She just
marches out the room. Mother of Tracy (age 9)

Blaming parents who punish their children for wetting the bed moves an
understanding of family process little further forward. By focusing only on
parents' responses to a situation the conditions which lead to their behaviour
can be all too easily ignored. As illustrated above, parents' misunderstanding
of their children's responses to criticism can lead to a self-perpetuating cycle
in which negative behaviours are continually evoked between and among
family members.

In those families where the parents said that they had adopted an attitude of
acceptance and tolerance this may have helped to ease the young person's
feelings of shame and helped to create a more supportive social environment
for the young person to learn the skill of becoming dry at night. However,
there was evidence that parents and young people sometimes saw situations
differently:

MR C: I don't bother about it. It's an illness you can't help, you can't do
anything about. So you've got to take it or leave it - like it or lump it - just
take it as it comes. You've got to take it - the things I've seen! - this is
nothing. So what?
CAROL: That's not what you say to me! You give me big lectures about it!
MR C: Yes, so what? It doesn't bother me, like. I just give you lectures
because you lie in it ... she just lies in it and doesn't tell anybody. That's
what gets me about it. Stepfather of Carol (age 17)

Carol had adopted an attitude of resigned helplessness and hopelessness.
Carol's apathy in the mornings was interpreted by her stepfather as a lack of
willingness to help herself in ways that she could control and she described
the worst thing about bed wetting as:

CAROL: ... getting shouted at, having to get up for a bath and changing my
bed, then getting slagged off. Carol (age 17)

Even in those families where the parents seemed to have adopted an
optimistic attitude towards the bed wetting, many young people had a
pessimistic view of their parents' evaluation of their behaviour. It may take no
more than an occasional disapproving glance at a wet bed by a parent to
reinforce the young person's belief that their bed wetting is regarded by them
as unacceptable behaviour.

In conclusion, while the interactions between family members appeared to

173

the researcher, as onlooker, to be reflexive, individuals within the family seemed to be seeing and interpreting situations in a linear fashion and from their own perspective, as illustrated above. As a consequence of this way of thinking parents seemed to perceive their own behaviour primarily as a response to the behaviour of the bed wetting child. For the most part they seemed to be quite unaware of the existence and consequences of mutual influence and their own contribution to the situations in which they found themselves.

A concept analysis of perceived helplessness and perceived control

Perceived helplessness appeared in many guises in the data and was at first identified as the central phenomenon or core concept in this study. Further analysis suggested that this concept was transcended by the concept of perceived control. This section begins by exploring the phenomenon of perceived helplessness, its antecedent conditions and its consequences. This is followed by a concept analysis of perceived control where this study's findings are briefly compared with the vast body of research into this construct which has been conducted in other settings.

Perceived helplessness

The causal conditions for perceived helplessness and feelings of shame experienced by young people in this study were identified as:

- past experience of repeated failure with treatment

- unrewarded effort

- the belief that most three year olds are able to be dry at night, which defines the task as easy, and

- negative evaluation of bed wetting by others.

Burns (1980) suggests that individuals behave according to their self conceptualisation, so that it becomes a self-fulfilling prophecy. The self image is validated by behaviour which in turn generates confirmatory feedback from others. A major consequence of feelings of shame and belief in helplessness is that many young people come to behave as though they are helpless. They may refuse to participate in treatment regimens suggested by others, or at best their participation is half-hearted. They do not sustain their efforts to become dry for long enough for the method to achieve the desired outcome. They are easily discouraged and interpret setbacks as confirmation that any initial success was due to chance, and their belief in their inability to influence the situation is reinforced. Furthermore their apathy is often construed by their parents as a lack of concern about the bed wetting and they may be punished for not making sufficient effort to help themselves. The result can be a cycle of helplessness involving both parents and young people. The situation is summarised in the axial coding diagram illustrated in Figure 5.10.

Establishing the sequence of events depicted in Figure 5.10 helped to account for many young people's attitudes towards bed wetting of resigned helplessness and hopelessness, which was characterised by both apathy and sadness.

Lazarus (1991) describes sadness as a negative emotion which is usually linked to loss, such as the death of a loved one, the failure of a central life value or role, or the loss of the positive regard of another person whose opinion is valued. He suggests that sadness is characterised by:

- irrevocable loss

- a sense of helplessness about restoration of the loss, and

- resignation rather than struggle.

Sadness, he suggests, indicates a move towards acceptance of and disengagement from the lost commitment. He suggests that emotional distress is actually attenuated when the individual "gives up" something that is perceived to be irrecoverable. In this sense giving up may serve an adaptive function. Futile endeavour is maladaptive.

Lazarus (1991) suggests that if the person does not perceive himself or herself to be completely helpless then other emotions are more likely in response to loss, such as anger, guilt or hope, which are associated with the initiation of restorative actions. While sadness is characterised by low engagement, as was seen in those young people who had adopted an attitude of resigned helplessness and hopelessness the emotions of anger, guilt or hope are accompanied by higher engagement in activities aimed at restoring what has been lost, in this case both bladder control and the self esteem associated with it.

Those young people who had adopted an attitude of optimistic pragmatism towards their bed wetting may have felt helpless to influence the situation at that time but they were not without hope that they would one day be dry.

A. CAUSAL CONDITIONS	1. Past experience of repeated failure with treatment methods, whether or not prescribed by health care professionals 2. Unrewarded effort 3. The belief that most 3 year olds are dry at night 4. Negative evaluation of bed wetting by others
B. PHENOMENON	**Perceived helplessness and feelings of shame** Young people who wet the bed come to believe that they cannot achieve their desired goal of becoming dry at night through their own efforts and that any dry nights that they do experience are due to chance. They feel ashamed at their lack of ability to do what a younger child can do.
C. CONTEXT	1. **Past experience of repeated failure** *The young person may have engaged in many methods in the past to attain night time continence and none of them has led to the achievement of the desired outcome* 2. **Unrewarded effort** *The young person wants to be dry at night but has achieved no more than the occasional dry night however hard he has tried in the past* 3. **The knowledge that most 3 year olds are dry at night** *A younger brother or sister may now be dry* 4. **Negative evaluation of the bed wetting by others** *The young person receives the message that he <u>ought</u> to be able to be dry at night from others within and outwith the household. The consistency with which the young person receives the negative meta message that his behaviour is both unacceptable and within his control contributes to the young person's feelings of shame and helplessness.*
D. INTERVENING CONDITIONS	1. **Parents may believe themselves to be helpless, feel helpless and behave as though they are helpless, from time to time** 2. **Health care professionals may believe themselves to be helpless, feel helpless and behave as though they are helpless, from time to time** *based on their past experience of repeated failure and unrewarded effort*

Figure 5.10   The use of a coding paradigm (axial coding) to explore the phenomenon of perceived helplessness, as experienced by many young people who wet the bed

176

<table>
<tr><td>

E. ACTION/
   INTERACTION
   STRATEGIES

</td><td>

Young people come to behave as though they are helpless

1. Young people do not sustain their efforts to become dry at night for long enough for the method to achieve the desired outcome because they do not expect it to be successful
2. They are easily discouraged and interpret setbacks in treatment efficacy as confirmation that any initial success was due to chance. Their belief in their own inability to influence the situation is reinforced by failure
3. They may refuse altogether to participate in treatment regimens suggested by others or at best participate half-heartedly

</td></tr>
<tr><td>

F. CONSEQUENCES

</td><td>

How parents and young people interpret and respond to each other's behaviour on "wet" mornings

1. Parents interpret the young person's behaviour as proof that:
   a. the young person is not concerned about wetting the bed, or won't face up to the problem
   b. the young person is not playing his part in helping the bed wetting to stop
2. The parents feel angry, frustrated, perhaps helpless
3. On finding that the young person has wet the bed the parents may:
   a. express their feelings of anger and frustration, verbally as well as non-verbally
   b. accuse the young person of not making the effort to be dry
4. The young people feel helpless and ashamed and may:
   a. reflect the parents' behaviour back to them on 'wet' mornings, or walk away from a confrontation
   b. distance themselves from the bed wetting by taking special care with their hygiene before leaving the house *(perhaps an end stage phenomenon is when they don't do this but actually lie awake in a wet bed, this could be the ultimate signal that the young person really has given up trying)*
5. The cycle of helplessness for both parents and the young people who wet the bed is self-perpetuating.

</td></tr>
</table>

Figure 5.10   Continued

In more than half of these cases their parents had been bed wetters and had become spontaneously dry so these young people knew from experience close to home that dry nights were possible. The message of Ian's parents to their son was characterised by hope for the future:

Mr I: We keep hoping that this is the time.
MRS I: We've told him that.
MR I: Ken, when he reaches a certain age, it's going to stop.

Father and mother of Ian (age 13)

Ian's mother had wet the bed herself until she was 11 years old.

It so happened that the two young people who were most angry about their bed wetting, Simon and Paul, had also taken the most responsibility for helping themselves to be dry and actually became dry shortly after their enrolment into the study. It is suggested that this attitude towards the bed wetting may have contributed to the outcome.

Ford (1992, p.137) describes anger as an energising emotion:

... anger and determination ... may be just what is needed to overcome seemingly intractable obstacles to goal attainment ... 'I'm mad as hell, and I'm not going to take it any more!'

Lazarus (1991, p.218) suggests that blame rather than mere accountability is crucial for anger:

To blame persons, rather than simply hold them accountable or responsible ... requires ... that we believe that they could have acted differently, that they had control over the offending action.

While anger is usually directed towards others it can be directed inwards, as is believed to have been the case for Simon and Paul, with the result that they redoubled their efforts to be dry. The fact that they were angry rather than sad about their bed wetting suggests that they had come to believe that they could exercise some control over the situation, that they could act differently. Paul's father described how his son's attitude towards his bed wetting changed from sadness to annoyance, which led to action:

MR P: ... its stymied him as far as going off and doing things - for a while - then he thought, 'nuts to it!' - you know - carried on - which is a great credit to him ... once he took control of himself - and you know, was saying 'I'm so frustrated by this, I must do something about it' and when he got to that stage it started to change. Because he was then feeling as though he was in control of himself and making his own decisions, and making his own mind up about it.

Father of Paul (age 13)

Perceived control

In the broadest sense, perceptions of control can be thought of as naive causal models individuals hold about how the world works: about the likely causes of desired and undesired events, about their own role in successes and failures, about the responsiveness of other people. ... People strive to experience control because humans have an innate need to be effective in interactions with the environment.

Skinner (1995) p.xvi-xvii

Five decades of research have established perceived control to be powerfully predictive of people's behaviour and motivation in many domains of life including: adaptation to chronic illness (Affleck et al, 1987; Braden, 1992; Hewlett, 1994; Watson et al, 1990); pain management (Arntz and Schmidt, 1989; Clements and Cummings, 1991; Walding, 1991); patient decision making (Fuchs, 1987; Kaplan, 1991); adjustment to ageing (Brandstaedter and Renner, 1990; Foy and Mitchell, 1990; Reich and Zautra, 1991); academic performance in school children (Patrick et al, 1993; Schmitz and Skinner, 1993; Skinner et al, 1988a,b), and coping with stress (Compas et al, 1991; Wannon, 1990).

This brief review of the concept of perceived control begins with an overview of four distinct yet interrelated constructs which have contributed to an understanding of a system of beliefs which transcends it, which is sometimes referred to as the competence system (Connell and Wellborn, 1991; Skinner, 1995). The four constructs are:

- locus of control (Rotter, 1966, 1975; Lefcourt, 1992)

- learned helplessness (Seligman, 1975; Abramson et al, 1978)

- causal attribution (Weiner, 1986, 1992), and

- self-efficacy (Bandura, 1989).

There are many other related concepts, such as Ford's (1992) concept of personal agency beliefs, which are incorporated into other theories of motivation. This brief review has been restricted to the concepts listed above because they have formed the basis of a great deal of research into the related constructs of perceived control, motivation and coping.

Locus of control In the original formulation of this theory Rotter (1966, p.1) describes two perspectives that individuals may have of their control over the outcomes of their actions:

> When a reinforcement is perceived by the subject as ... not being entirely contingent upon his action, then ... it is typically perceived as the result of luck, chance, fate, as under the control of powerful others, or as unpredictable ... When the event is interpreted in this way by an individual, we have labelled this as a belief in *external control*. If the person perceives that the event is contingent upon his own behaviour or his own relatively permanent characteristics, we have termed this a belief in *internal control*.

Locus of control is said to influence success or failure through its effects on effort expenditure and persistence in the attainment of a goal. It was proposed that locus of control influences the individual's expectancy of success in any situation. An internal locus of control has been said to predict a more positive outcome than an external locus of control in a variety of situations (Strickland, 1989; Lefcourt, 1992). Hundreds of studies have involved the measurement of locus of control but Ford (1992) suggests that this literature is filled with results that are anomalous or hard to interpret. He warns of the dangers of assuming that predictive precision is achievable using such a global measure of the perceived control construct as no account is taken of the influence of context.

In a critique of locus of control as a construct Skinner (1995, p.4) comments:

> ... it is easy to assume that an individual's generalized sense of control constitutes a stable, enduring, cross-situational trait-like predisposition ... Studies in which individuals are labelled as 'internals' and 'externals' contribute to this impression. In current conceptualizations, however, perceived control is usually considered a flexible set of inter-related beliefs that are organized around interpretations of prior interactions in specific domains.

Skinner suggests that an individual's perceived control is not a fixed and enduring personal quality but involves a set of personally constructed beliefs which can be changed in the light of new experience, even if a great deal of contradictory evidence is required to alter them.

Locus of control was not measured in the participants in this study but a clear impression was gained from talking with both young people and their parents that the young people's perceived lack of control over their bladder function at night was regarded by most as a very situation-specific phenomenon. There was, however, a small group of young people, such as Carol and Stephen, who behaved as though their predominant tendency was towards a belief in external control and the attitude of these young people to their bed wetting was one of resigned helplessness and hopelessness.

Learned helplessness The theory of learned helplessness has undergone several revisions since it was originally proposed in the early 1970s. The original studies examined the links between non-contingency and subsequent cognitive, behavioural and motivational deficits. Based on the findings of experiments involving rats and dogs (Richter, 1958; Seligman and Maier, 1967) the central proposition was that when people experience aversive events that occur independently of their own responses they learn that they are helpless and this belief in helplessness becomes more generalised. When people who have learned that they are helpless in one situation are placed in situations where some control is possible, it is suggested that they continue to behave as though they are helpless, that is they are passive and do not seek out the control that is possible.

Learned helplessness has been implicated in some forms of depression (Abramson et al, 1989; Hiroto and Seligman, 1975; Seligman, 1975; Wetzel, 1994) and has been reported as an outcome for both women and children following years of physical or sexual abuse (Blair, 1986; Kelley, 1986).

Since its original inception the theory has been revised. According to Abramson et al (1978) following experiences of non-contingency individuals seek to explain the cause. The attribution for response-outcome non contingency can be classified on three dimensions of causality: locus, stability and globality. Stability leads to chronicity, globality is a measure of cross-situational generality and locus affects the individual's self esteem.

It is not known whether young people's experience of helplessness in the context of their bed wetting (which in some cases had been experienced for many years), had affected their perception of their control in other situations or whether and to what extent it may have contributed to more general feelings of resigned helplessness and hopelessness, where these were in evidence.

Causal attributions Weiner (1986, 1992) has developed a theory of motivation based on causal attribution. He proposes that when something negative or unexpected happens people ask themselves why. The causes to which individuals attribute events can be placed along a number of dimensions which include: internality, stability, controllability and intentionality. These dimensions predict many important outcomes such as emotions, behaviour and the motivation to act.

When an individual attributes a successful outcome to their own ability, it leads to enhanced self esteem, high expectations of success in the future and persistence with the activity in the mean time. When an individual attributes lack of success to low ability, as a result of persistent failure in the past, in spite of effort, the individual experiences low self esteem, feels helpless, expects failure in the future and is unlikely to persist with the activity. This is reminiscent of the behaviour of many young people in this study who believed themselves to be helpless to stop their bed wetting.

Weiner's attribution theory has found applications in many domains ranging from scholastic achievement and achievement in the work place to recovery from: rape; life-threatening illness, and traumatic accidents (Skinner, 1995). Causal attributions can influence motivation in powerful ways by altering an individual's expectations in relation to capability of achievement in the future.

Self efficacy According to Bandura (1989) an individual's emotions and behaviour are a reflection of the interaction of self efficacy and outcome expectancy. Effective action is most likely when an individual has a positive judgement of his self efficacy and a high expectation of a positive outcome. An individual who believes that his self efficacy is low and a positive outcome is unlikely is, by contrast, likely to be apathetic and resigned. If a person with a belief in his own low self-efficacy believes that others do enjoy the benefits of their efforts then Bandura suggests that the result is self devaluation and despondency. This is akin to the situation for many bed wetters who believe that they themselves have no control over the situation which can be controlled by most three year olds. They believe that the task is easy and should be readily achievable because most pre-school infants can achieve it. Bandura (1989) suggests that an individual's expectation of success in a given situation may be enough to create that success and even to blunt the impact of minor failures. The illusion of control may be adaptive if it leads to positive emotions such as optimism. This theme is explored further in Chapter 6.

A new conceptualisation of perceived control Based on research into perceived control and achievement in school children (e.g. Skinner et al, 1988a,b; Schmitz and Skinner, 1993) and drawing upon different aspects of perceived control highlighted by studies of the related constructs of locus of control, learned helplessness, causal attribution and self efficacy described above, Skinner (1995) has proposed a new conceptualisation of perceived control. She distinguishes between three kinds of belief:

- control beliefs - which refer to generalised expectancies about the extent to which the self can produce desired or prevent undesired events

- strategy (means-end) beliefs - which refer to generalised expectancies about the extent to which certain means are sufficient conditions for the production of ends (outcomes), and

- capacity (agency) beliefs - which refer to generalised expectancies about the extent to which the self possesses or has access to certain means.

Skinner proposes that these three belief sets function in the regulation and interpretation of action. Strategy and capacity beliefs are involved in the evaluation and interpretation of performance. They are both used in the individual's attempt to understand the meaning of successes and failures and are themselves influenced by performance outcome. Control beliefs are a combination of strategy and capacity beliefs. Control beliefs are analogous to performance expectations and success estimation.

According to Skinner's (1995, p.35-36) conceptualisation, strategy and capacity beliefs are independent:

A person can be high on capacity ('I have all the means') and still report low strategy beliefs ('But none of the means produce any outcomes'). Or a person can be high on strategy beliefs ('There are lots of means that lead to outcomes') but still perceive him - or herself - as lacking in capacity ('But I don't have any of them').

Strategy beliefs are about "what it takes to ... " while capacity beliefs relate to the individual's perception of himself as "having what it takes to ...". Strategy beliefs have a parallel in the construct of locus of control and include beliefs about whether the outcome is dependent upon: effort, ability, powerful others or luck. Skinner et al (1988a,b) used these dimensions to develop profiles of perceived control which they postulated would predict engagement versus disaffection in the academic domain.

Skinner et al (1990) found that children's engagement was positively related to control beliefs and capacity beliefs for effort and ability, in the way predicted and was undermined by strategy beliefs relating to luck. The highest levels of engagement were found among children who reported that effort was an effective means and that they had the capacity to exert effort.

It is suggested in Chapter 6 that similar research into young people's control beliefs could be helpful in predicting which young people are likely to persist with treatment for their bed wetting for long enough for it to be effective. It is suggested, however, that prolonged engagement is also likely to be strongly influenced by parents' own control beliefs as most young people are likely to require a measure of help and support during this time.

In seeking an answer to the question: 'How do individual differences in perceived control develop?' Skinner (1995) puts forward a theory based on the assumption articulated by Seligman in 1975 in relation to learned helplessness, namely that control beliefs and their consequences can create a self-perpetuating cycle:

> Individuals who believe they have control act in ways that make success more likely and so confirm their initial high expectations of control. Furthermore, their sustained engagement in challenging tasks is likely to lead to the development of actual competence over time. In contrast, individuals who do not believe they can influence outcomes act in ways that forfeit opportunities for exerting control. Over time, through their passivity and avoidance of difficult tasks, they forgo the development of new competencies. Individual differences in developmental trajectories of both subjective control and objective competence will result.
>
> Skinner (1995) p.xvii

The challenge for health care professionals is to foster in young people who wet the bed, and their parents, a belief that some control over the situation is possible (Chapter 6).

Summary

Most young people are sad and ashamed about wetting the bed and want it to stop but they vary widely in their belief in their own capacity to influence the situation and in their optimism about what the future holds.

Young people learn to feel ashamed of their bed wetting because of the negative evaluation of this behaviour by others, both within and outwith the household. They define the task as "easy" because they believe that most three year olds can achieve it. As a result of past experience of repeated failure to become dry at night, however hard they have tried, they attribute their own lack of success in this task to lack of ability. The threat posed to their self esteem by the censure of others causes many young people to try to hide their "deficiency" from others and to avoid situations which might lead to the discovery of their secret.

When a young person is blamed for wetting the bed the young person's feelings of humiliation and shame are reinforced because they have failed to live up to an ego-ideal and have disappointed another person or other persons whose approbation matters to them. As a result the young person experiences a further loss of control, an increasing sense of powerlessness and motivational inhibition. This is often interpreted by parents as a lack of concern. The young person is blamed for lack of effort and the cycle can become self perpetuating.

In situations where the young person is blamed and the bed wetting moves up the family's agenda, tension relating to bed wetting may increase as the young person's belief in his capacity to influence the situation declines, making the attainment of the desired goal less likely. The widespread practice by parents and others of blaming young people who wet the bed is therefore counter productive.

The implications of this study's findings for practice are explored in Chapter 6. This includes a discussion of how young people, their parents and indeed health care professionals can increase their belief in their capacity to influence a situation where the treatment process for bed wetting is controllable but where a rapid and successful outcome cannot be guaranteed.

6 Implications for practice and possible directions for further research

The findings of this study have a number of implications for practice, many of which could form the basis for further research.

As outlined in the literature review, the aetiology of bed wetting and how best to treat it are still matters of considerable debate (Chapter 1). The data presented in Chapter 3 and elsewhere suggest that understanding more about the natural history of the acquisition of nocturnal bladder control could be a fruitful line of inquiry.

The focus of this study and this chapter is, however, on the family as the context within which bed wetting is experienced and treated. The chapter begins by outlining the conditions suggested by the data to be required to maximise the likelihood of a successful treatment outcome. The concept of a family's readiness to engage in treatment is explored. Some ways of enhancing young people's, parents' and health care professionals' sense of competence, in a situation where many individuals have come to believe themselves to be helpless, are described. The implications of this study for service organisation are discussed.

Some conditions required to maximise the likelihood of a successful outcome to treatment

It is strongly suggested by the data that the following conditions (C1-C5) may need to be met for the young person to have the best chance of achieving dry nights as the result of an intervention:

$$C1 + C2 + C3 + C4 + C5$$

C1 = both the young person and the parents want the bed wetting to stop

C2 = both the young person and the parents believe that the achievement of dry nights is contingent upon their efforts and that they are capable of making the effort required

C3 = the goal of achieving dry nights is not out-competed by more pressing priorities on the family's agenda for action

C4 = the family gain access to a treatment method appropriate to the young person's needs, which is within both the parents' and the young person's capability

C5 = the family have easy and rapid access to professional support and help especially if they experience equipment failure, apparent lack of progress or the young person or the parents cease to believe in treatment.

It is suggested that in the absence of any one of these conditions it is unlikely that any treatment prescribed by health care professionals will be sustained for long enough to stand a good chance of success. These conditions were arrived at empirically but they are congruent with Ford's (1992, p.69) scheme for classifying the processes which contribute to goal achievement:

$$\text{Achievement/Competence} = \frac{\text{Motivation x Skill}}{\text{Biology}} \text{ x Responsive Environment}$$

Ford suggests that achievement is the result of a motivated, skilful and biologically capable person interacting with a responsive environment, which facilitates, or at least does not excessively impede progress towards a goal. However Ford (1992, p.124) suggests that it is not enough to have a goal in mind and the objective skills and circumstances to achieve it:

> People must also *believe* that they have the capabilities and opportunities needed to achieve their goal. Indeed, such beliefs are often more fundamental than the actual skills and circumstances they represent in the sense that they can motivate people to create opportunities and acquire capabilities they do not yet possess ...[quoting Kolligan and Sternberg, 1990]: 'At all points in the life cycle it is one's construal of reality, rather than reality itself, that most accurately predicts self-concepts, goals, academic performance, and overall mental health'.

It is suggested in the conditions (C1-C5) listed above, that capability beliefs are necessary for a successful outcome to an intervention but they are not sufficient to ensure a successful outcome. As well as not being out-competed (C3), it is suggested that the families require to be provided with a responsive and supportive environment by health care professionals.

In the present study the parents clearly felt that most health care professionals had little to offer them, although their intention to be facilitative was rarely questioned (Chapter 4). This situation is not helped by the lack of certainty amongst professionals about the aetiology of bed wetting and how best to treat it. The need to enhance health care professionals' sense of competence in the context of the management of bed wetting is touched upon later in the present chapter.

Assessing the family's readiness to engage in treatment

The data from this study suggest that most parents believe that they are helpless, feel helpless, and behave as though they are helpless to influence the young person's bed wetting from time to time. In some cases this belief is accompanied by feelings of hopelessness. It has also been shown that many young people come to believe that they are helpless, feel helpless and behave as though they are helpless to stop wetting the bed (Chapter 5). A relationship between the parent's and the young person's perception of themselves as helpless to influence the situation and the likelihood of the family taking and persisting with action to encourage the bed wetting to stop is proposed in the form of a conditional matrix (Figure 6.1).

It is suggested that the testing of the hypotheses depicted in Figure 6.1 could be a fruitful line for research. The two components of perceived control, namely strategy beliefs and capacity beliefs, proposed by Skinner et al (1988a,b), could be tested using a form of the Perceptions of Control Questionnaire (Skinner, 1995), modified for the domain of bed wetting.

If it is confirmed by such research that the combination of the parents' and the young person's perception of control is predictive of their engagement in treatment, and their persistence or otherwise with it in the light of setbacks, it would seem prudent to assess these parameters prior to prescribing any treatment regimen. If either the young person or the parents, or both, are assessed as perceiving themselves to be helpless, it is suggested that the first priority should be to attempt to enhance these individuals' beliefs in their own competence. Some strategies for enhancing the individual's belief in competence are proposed in the next section.

	Young person, who wets the bed, believes that he or she is HELPLESS	
	YES	NO
Parent believes that he or she is HELPLESS — **YES**	**NO ACTION** No action taken by parent or young person to stop the bed wetting	**ACTION UNLIKELY** While young person may believe that taking action could lead to more dry nights, action is unlikely as parents are the gatekeepers to resources needed to take action
Parent believes that he or she is HELPLESS — **NO**	**ACTION MAY BE INITIATED BUT IS UNLIKELY TO BE SUSTAINED** Parents may attempt to initiate a treatment regimen but young person's co-operation and commitment is at best half-hearted as their expectancy of success is low	**BEST CHANCE THAT ACTION WILL BE BOTH INITIATED AND SUSTAINED** Parent(s) and young person actively engage together in methods to stop the bed wetting - UNLESS the resolution of the young person's bed wetting is out-competed on the family's agenda by more pressing priorities within the family at the time

Figure 6.1 **The hypothesised relationship between the parent's and the young person's belief in helplessness and the likelihood of action being taken to encourage the bed wetting to stop (once the bed wetting has been identified by them both as a problem)**

189

It is shown in this study that the active treatment of the young person's bed wetting can be out-competed by other priorities on the family's agenda for action (Chapter 4). Assessing the appropriateness of the timing of any intervention, with families, in relation to other family priorities at the time could be of particular importance in ensuring that the optimum time is chosen to embark on any treatment regimen which is likely to require the prolonged co-operation of all the family.

For treatment to be successful it is axiomatic that the young person should desire the goal which is to be striven for. There is evidence presented in this study to suggest that a small minority of young people may gain some secondary benefits from bed wetting. This may be associated with a poor relationship with one or both parents. Careful questioning of the young person on his own and of the parents may help to identify such cases, which may not be obvious to a health care professional who does not know the family well. It may be that the family dynamics are assessed as being so unconducive to the provision of a supportive environment for the young person to learn the skills of becoming dry at night that the first step in treatment may need to be some form of family therapy to improve communication and to foster positive mutual regard and empathy between family members, as well as to enhance the family's collective problem solving skills.

Enhancing a belief in competence among young people, their parents and health care professionals

> Tasks of 'just manageable difficulty', which are replete with unsuccessful attempts, are the natural playground for the operation of the competence system, and dealing with them provides learning as well as joy and satisfaction. However, prolonged unpredictability and uncontrollability overwhelm the competence system and, when crystallized as a general sense of incompetence or non-contingency, prevent it from functioning optimally in response to challenges.   Skinner (1995) p.136

The need for competence is considered by Skinner to be an innate and universal human need. Competence in this context refers to the contingency between behaviours and outcomes and is the extent to which a person feels capable of producing desired and preventing undesired events. Its opposite is non-competence, that is helplessness.

Many examples of young people and their parents perceiving themselves to be helpless to influence the bed wetting are given in this monograph. A belief in competence can be enhanced among young people and their parents when they are provided with opportunities for exercising and experiencing effective control.

Exhortations to make more effort may be counter-productive

In situations where individuals already perceive themselves to be doing badly, emphasising the effectiveness of effort may lead them to feel even more incompetent. They may further doubt their own abilities, stop trying and experience increased negative self evaluation. It is suggested that this is what is happening in the cases of those young people who are being told by their parents (usually their fathers) that they could be dry if only they tried harder (Chapter 5).

In the academic domain this phenomenon has been described by Covington and Omelich (1979, p.169) as "the double-edged sword" of effort. Failure in spite of high effort expenditure is attributed to low ability. Covington and Omelich (1985) suggest in the school setting that given a choice between being judged lazy and being judged stupid, most people prefer to be seen as lazy. It may be that young people who wet the bed would rather be judged lazy than incapable of performing a task perceived to be within the control of a three year old, particularly as they grow older. This, combined with their knowledge from experience that effort is futile, may account for many young people's disengagement or at best half-heartedness when engaged in treatment. Half-hearted action only increases the experience of failure, leading to frustration and perhaps to feelings of hopelessness.

Creating opportunities where effective control is possible

It is suggested that enhancing a belief in competence among young people and their parents can be facilitated when opportunities are created for them to experience effective control. In the case of bed wetting this can involve exercising control over the treatment process, although the outcome cannot be guaranteed, and minimising the effects of the practical consequences of bed wetting.

One way of increasing the experience of effective control, come upon serendipitously in this study, is to encourage young people to keep a truthful record of their wet and dry nights which is not linked to any reward for dry nights. Instead it is suggested that parents reward only the truthful and timely keeping of the record. Many parents found from their own experience that offering rewards for dry nights put too much pressure on the young person, with the result that the number of wet nights increased. In this study several young people came to see that dry nights were possible through the keeping of the diary and the success was attributed by them to their own efforts and not to chance. In a sense, whether the increase in the number of dry nights achieved was, in fact, due to chance does not matter. The individual's perception that the outcome was contingent on their efforts is what matters as this can lead to increased engagement with a difficult task, enhanced self esteem and optimism for the future.

If it is decided that the circumstances are right for some form of behavioural training such as a bedside or body-worn alarm, the young person should be rewarded for actively engaging in the method and keeping an accurate and timely record rather than for achieving dry nights *per se*. More dry nights may of themselves be sufficient motivation for the young person to continue with treatment once the outcome is seen to be contingent on effort.

Until the young person becomes reliably dry, it may be helpful for parents to encourage young people to take more responsibility for managing the practical consequences of the wet beds, perhaps with a simple system of rewards or a points system leading to a special treat. This could have the added benefit of reducing the work load for the parents and the tension for everyone within the household in the mornings. The appropriateness of this approach would need to be carefully discussed with the parents. Some parents may feel that the young person should play their part in the practicalities without the need for any tangible reward. Consistent praise may well be sufficient to convey to the young person the message: "We appreciate your help with this task" and to foster a sense of mutual co-operation. What is important is that the management of the practicalities is not portrayed as a punishment: "You wet the bed, you clear it up!"

Encouraging realistic expectations

There is evidence that the most adaptive control beliefs are realistic ones (Wannon, 1990). Malone-Lee (1992) suggests, in the context of bed wetting, that it is important not to raise false expectations of the likelihood of a successful outcome from treatment. There were many examples of unrealistic reassurance having been given to individuals in this study, as mentioned for example by Anthony:

ANTHONY: Everyone gave me, like, an age when it would stop at. I thought, 'Oh great, it will just stop overnight when I'm that age', and of course it never did.   Anthony (age 16)

It is important for health care professionals to acknowledge to families that the attainment of night time bladder control is not an easy task for some young people and it is outwith their conscious control in most cases. The data suggest that one of the most important things that health care professionals working with families can do is to encourage parents to create a supportive social and emotional climate within the home for the young person to learn the skill of becoming dry at night. This involves parents in accepting the young person as he or she is, acknowledging all the young person's attempts at self help, focusing on any positive gains, however small and avoiding blame.

If treatment fails it is important that the message is conveyed to families that this is not the fault of the young person or their parents if they have engaged in the treatment conscientiously, as the reasons why some young people respond to certain treatments while others do not are far from certain (Chapter 1). Asking families to repeat treatment regimes which they do not believe in is doomed to failure (Chapter 4).

When engaged in a difficult task it is clearly maladaptive to interpret each setback as evidence of lack of ability, yet this is what most young people quite understandably seem to do. In challenging situations where active engagement is essential, people can maintain their own engagement by regulating their action, through such means as intentional self-encouragement, boosting determination, and optimism. Active engagement is facilitated by bolstering feelings of effectiveness and looking for contingencies but these coping strategies are almost certainly beyond the capacity of younger children. There are many books available on techniques to enhance "positive thinking" but positive thinking, on its own, is not enough. The task for health care professionals is to provide a supportive and responsive environment to ensure that family members' efforts stand the best chance of being rewarded and to encourage parents to do the same.

Enhancing a sense of competence among health care professionals

Many of the principles outlined above are equally applicable to health care professionals. The aim is to encourage health care professionals to engage with families in a difficult task for long enough for success to be achieved, to have realistic expectations and to be able to handle setbacks without resorting to disengagement. It is suggested that the confidence of health care professionals in their ability to help families could be enhanced by the availability of evidence based clinical protocols which would help them to give care known by them to meet "best practice" standards. Even the illusion of control could be adaptive, as it could motivate professionals to acquire capabilities that they do not yet possess through prolonged engagement with a challenging task.

Implications for service organisation

As this study shows, many professionals may become involved in helping families where one or more children wet the bed, including: health visitors; general practitioners; school nurses; continence nurse advisers; paediatricians; urologists; clinical medical officers; psychiatrists; clinical psychologists and social workers.

Wright and Leahey (1993, p.27) stress the importance of assessing a health problem at all system levels, and then intervening at the system level "with the greatest leverage for change". If a pathological problem is suspected at the organ system level, a specialist opinion from a urologist may be pivotal to ensuring that the most appropriate care is initiated. If the problem is assessed as being exacerbated by poor interpersonal relationships within the family, then the situation may, in some cases, require the intervention of a specialist in family therapy. It is suggested, however, that for most monosymptomatic bed wetters the management of the bed wetting is well within the remit of the members of the primary health care team.

Enuresis clinics are being set up and evaluated in many parts of the UK and abroad (Chisholm, 1995; Larsen et al, 1992; Vermaak, 1992) and can provide a valuable service, but it is suggested that unless a member of the primary health care team is involved with the clinic the context within which the bed wetting is being managed by the family may be lost sight of.

When working with pre-school children the health visitor is particularly likely to discover the family's "secret" and to be in a position to give practical advice and support to the family as a whole. Often the health visitor acts as the gatekeeper to more specialist services, via the general practitioner.

It is, however, unrealistic to expect that all health visitors will have the necessary specialist knowledge to act effectively. There is evidence to suggest that some health visitors and school nurses do not feel confident about their abilities to help families with the management of bed wetting (Paterson, 1993). In Paterson's study, a number of health visitors commented that they had received no formal education or training in this area. To quote one of Paterson's respondents "we need more training, more equipment and more expertise" (p.423). It is therefore suggested that health visitors need to be supported in this role and to receive appropriate in-service training and opportunities for up dating (Chisholm, 1995; ERIC, 1993).

The establishment of inter-disciplinary evidence based clinical protocols for assessment and treatment and the development of explicit referral criteria could increase the probability of the family gaining access to the most appropriate help. Guidelines on minimum standards of practice are already in existence (Morgan, 1993) and could be built upon.

Summary

It is shown in this study that parents and young people are likely to enter into clinical relationships with pre-conceived ideas about the causes of the bed wetting and the young person's control over the situation. In many cases these views are likely to be at variance with the views of professionals. It is suggested that a difference between lay and professional viewpoints can lead to failures of intervention, especially when family members regard the treatment suggestions of health care professionals to be ill-conceived. Failure of professionals to assess and take cognisance of the responsiveness, or otherwise, of the social environment within which their treatments are to be conducted may also lead to treatment failure. Understanding the family's perspective enables a dialogue to be engaged in which takes account of the reality of the family's circumstances, including family members' beliefs, capabilities and access to resources.

Appendix A
Summary of contextual data relating to each family

Pseudonym of the young person who wet the bed	Age of young person	Parents currently living within the household				Relative deprivation of the electoral ward where the family lives[b]			Parent's experience of bed wetting		
		Natural mother	Natural father	Step father	Mother's male partner	Most affluent quartile	Inter-mediate quartiles	Least affluent quartile	Mother herself	Mother's sibling	Natural father himself
Carol	17	✓			✓			✓	✓	NK	✓
Anthony	16	✓	✓				✓		x	x	x
Peter	15	✓		✓		✓			x	✓	✓
Roger	14	✓	✓					✓	x	x	x
Paul	13	✓	✓				✓		✓	x	✓
Ian	13	✓	✓				✓		✓	✓	x
Sarah	11	✓	✓				✓		✓	✓	x
Jennifer	9	✓						✓	x	x	x
Alison	9	✓		✓				✓	x	✓	x
Tracy	9	✓				✓			x	x	x
William	9	✓			✓		✓		x	✓	x

Name										
Michelle	8	✓		✓			✓		x	✓	x
Simon	8	✓		✓		✓			x	x	x
Stephen[a]	8	✓					✓		✓	✓	✓
John[a]	8	✓					✓		✓	✓	✓
Michael	8	✓	✓			✓			x	x	x
Shelly	7	✓	✓					✓	✓	x	x
Martin	6	✓	✓				✓		x	x	x
Gary	5	✓	✓					✓	x	x	x
Lisa	4	✓	✓					✓	x	x	x

Notes: ✓ = YES   x = NO   NK = not known   [a] twins   [b] see Chapter 3

References

Abramovitch, I.B. & Abramovitch, H.H. (1989) Enuresis in cross cultural perspective: a comparison of training for elimination control in three Israeli ethnic groups. *Journal of Social Psychology*, **129(1)**, 47-56.

Abrams, P., Blaivas, J.G., Stanton, S.L. & Andersen, J.T. (1988) The standardisation of terminology of lower urinary tract function. *Scandinavian Journal of Urology and Nephrology.Supplementum*, **114**, 5-19.

Abramson, L.Y., Metalsky, G.I. & Alloy, L.B. (1989) Hopelessness depression: a theory-based subtype of depression. *Psychological Review*, **96(2)**, 358-372.

Abramson, L.Y., Seligman, M.E.P. & Teasdale, J.D. (1978) Learned helplessness in humans: critique and reformulation. *Journal of Abnormal Psychology*, **87(1)**, 49-74.

Affleck, G., Tennen, H., Pfeiffer, C. & Fifield, J. (1987) Appraisals of control and predictability in adapting to a chronic disease. *Journal of Personality and Social Psychology*, **53(2)**, 273-279.

Agar, M. (1993) The right brain strikes back. *Using computers in qualitative research* (ed. by N.G. Fielding and R.M. Lee), p.181-194. Sage, London.

Amato, P.R. (1986a) Marital conflict, the parent-child relationship, and child self-esteem. *Family Relations*, **35**, 403-410.

Amato, P.R. (1986b) Father involvement and the self-esteem of children and adolescents. *Australian Journal of Sex, Marriage and Family*, **7**, 6-16.

Amato, P.R. & Ochiltree, G. (1987) Interviewing children about their families: a note on data quality. *Journal of Marriage and the Family*, **49**, 669-675.

Ambrosini, P.J. (1993) Antidepressant treatments in children and adolescents: II Anxiety, physical and behavioural disorders. *Journal of the American Academy of Child and Adolescent Psychiatry*, **32(3)**, 483-493.

Anderson, N.L.R. (1987) Computer use and nursing research: computer-assisted analysis of textual field note data. *Western Journal of Nursing Research*, **9(4)**, 626-630.

Anderson, R. & Bury, M. (1988) *Living with chronic illness: the experience of patients and their families*, Unwin Hyman, London.

Arntz, A. & Schmidt, A.J.M. (1989) Perceived control and the experience of pain. *Stress, personal control and health* (ed. by A. Steptoe and A. Appels), p.131-161. John Wiley, Brussels.

Azrin, N.H., Sneed, T.J. & Fox, R.M. (1974) Dry bed training: rapid elimination of childhood enuresis. *Behaviour Research and Therapy*, **12**, 147-156.

Azrin, N.H. & Thienes, P.M. (1978) Rapid elimination of enuresis by intensive learning without a conditioning apparatus. *Behavior Therapy*, **9**, 342-354.

Bakwin, H. (1973) The genetics of enuresis. *Bladder control and enuresis* (ed. by I. Kolvin, R.C. MacKeith and S.R. Meadow), p.73-77. William Heinemann Medical Books, London.

Bandura, A. (1989) Human agency in social cognitive theory. *American Psychologist*, **44(9)**, 1175-1184.

Barker, P.J. (1991) Interview. *The research process in nursing* (ed. by D.F.S. Cormack), Blackwell Scientific Publications, Oxford.

Baron, R.A. & Byrne, D. (1994) *Social psychology: understanding human interaction*, Allyn and Bacon, London.

Barry, J. (1988) Night-time despair. *Nursing Times*, **84 (12)**, 82-85.

Baumarind, D. (1991) The influence of parenting style on adolescent competence and substance use. *Journal of Early Adolescence*, **1**, 56-95.

Becker, P.H. (1993) Common pitfalls in published grounded theory research. *Qualitative Health Research*, **3 (2)**, 254-260.

Bell, J.M. (1995) Avoiding isomorphism: a call for a different view. *Journal of Family Nursing*, **1(1)**, 5-7.

Belsky, J. (1981) Early human experience: a family perspective. *Developmental Psychology*, **17**, 3-23.

Belsky, J. (1990) Parental and non parental child care and children's socioemotional development: a decade in review. *Journal of Marriage and the Family*, **52**, 885-903.

Belsky, J., Youngblade, L., Rovine, M. & Volling, B. (1991) Patterns of marital change and parent-child interaction. *Journal of Marriage and the Family*, **53**, 487-498.

Bernstein, D.A., Roy, E.J., Srull, T.K. & Wickens, C.D. (1991) *Psychology*, Houghton Mifflin, Boston.

Biller, H.B. (1993) *Fathers and families: paternal factors in child development*, Auburn House, Westport, CT.

Blackwell, C. (1989) *A guide to the treatment of enuresis for professionals*, Enuresis Resource and Information Centre, Bristol.

Blackwell, C. (1992) Investigation of the acquisition of nocturnal dryness. *Papers from the second national conference of the Enuresis Resource and Information Centre (1991): a comprehensive approach to nocturnal enuresis* (ed. by P. Dobson), p.45-50. Enuresis Resource and Information Centre, Bristol.

Blackwell, C.L. (1995) *A guide to the treatment of enuresis for professionals*, Northumberland Clinical Psychology Service (available via Enuresis Resource and Information Centre, Bristol).

Blair, K.A. (1986) The battered woman: is she a silent victim? *Nurse Practitioner*, **11(6)**, 38-44.

Blomfield, J.M. & Douglas, J.M.B. (1956) Bed wetting prevalence among children aged 4 - 7 years. *Lancet*, **1**, 850-853.

Bloom, D.A., Seeley, W.W., Ritchey, M.L. & McGuire, E.J. (1993) Toilet habits and continence in children: an opportunity sampling in search of normal parameters. *Journal of Urology*, **149**, 1087-1090.

Bollard, J. & Nettlebeck, T. (1982) A component analysis of dry bed training for treatment for bed wetting. *Behaviour Research and Therapy*, **20**, 383-390.

Bollard, J. & Nettelbeck, T. (1989) *Bedwetting: a treatment manual for professional staff*, Chapman and Hall, London.

Borstelmann, L.J. (1983) Children before psychology: ideas about children from antiquity to the late 1800s. *Handbook of child psychology: Volume 1 history, theory and methods* (ed. by W. Kessen), p.1-40. Wiley, New York.

Bose, B. (1992) The attitudes of different social and ethnic groups to bedwetting: a review of the literature. *Papers from the second national conference of the Enuresis Resource and Information Centre (1991): a comprehensive approach to nocturnal enuresis* (ed. by P. Dobson), p.14-18. Enuresis Resource and Information Centre, Bristol.

Braden, C.J. (1992) Description of learned response to chronic illness: depressed vs nondepressed self-help class participants. *Public Health Nursing*, **9(2)**, 103-108.

Brandtstaedter, J. & Renner, G. (1990) Tenacious goal pursuit and flexible goal adjustment: explication and age-related analysis of assimilative and accommodative strategies of coping. *Psychology and Aging*, **5(1)**, 58-67.

Briere, J.N. (1992) *Child abuse trauma: theory and treatment of the lasting effects*, Sage, Newbury Park, CA.

Broderick, C.B. (1993) *Understanding family process: basics of family systems theory*, Sage, Newbury Park, CA.

Bronfenbrenner, U. (1986) Ecology of the family as a context for human development: research perspectives. *Developmental Psychology*, **22**, 723-742.

Buchan, D. (1994) Folk tradition and folk medicine in Scotland: the writings of David Rorie. *Canongate Academic, Edinburgh*, p.108.

Bunton, R., Murphy, S. & Bennett, P. (1991) Theories of behavioural change and their use in health promotion: some neglected areas. *Health Education Research*, **6(2)**, 153-162.

Burghes, L. (1994) *Lone parenthood and family disruption: the outcomes for children*, Family Policy Studies Centre, London.

Burgio, K.L., Matthews, K.A. & Engel, T. (1991) Prevalence, incidence and correlates of urinary incontinence in healthy, middle-aged women. *Journal of Urology*, **146(5)**, 1255-1259.

Burnand, P. (1989) *Counselling skills for health professionals*, Chapman and Hall, London.

Burns, R.B. (1980) *Essential psychology for students and professionals in the health and social services*, M T P Press, Lancaster.

Burr, W.R. & Klein, S.R. (1994) *Re-examining family stress: new theory and research*, Sage, Thousand Oaks, CA.

Butler, N.R. & Golding, J. (1986) *From birth to five: a study of Britain's five year olds*, Pergamon Press, Oxford.

Butler, R.J. (1987) *Nocturnal enuresis: psychological perspectives*, Wright, Bristol.

Butler, R.J. (1991) Establishment of working definitions in nocturnal enuresis. *Archives of Disease in Childhood*, **66**, 267-271.

Butler, R.J. (1993a) *Nocturnal enuresis: a manual of treatment methods*, Department of Psychology Highroyds Hospital, Menston.

Butler, R.J. (1993b) *Enuresis resource pack: charts, questionnaires and information to assist professionals*, The Enuresis Resource and Information Centre, Bristol.

Butler, R.J. (1994) *Nocturnal enuresis: the child's experience*, Butterworth Heinemann, Oxford.

Butler, R.J. & Brewin, C.R. (1986) Maternal views of nocturnal enuresis. *Health Visitor*, **59(7)**, 207-209.

Butler, R.J., Brewin, C.R. & Forsythe, W.I. (1986) Maternal attributions and tolerance for nocturnal enuresis. *Behaviour Research and Therapy*, **24(3)**, 307-312.

Butler, R.J., Brewin, C.R. & Forsythe, W.I. (1988) A comparison of two approaches to the treatment of nocturnal enuresis and the prediction of effectiveness using pre-treatment variables. *Journal of Child Psychology and Psychiatry and Applied Disciplines*, **29**, 501-509.

Butler, R.J., Forsythe, W.I. & Robertson, J. (1990) The body-worn alarm in the treatment of childhood enuresis. *British Journal of Clinical Practice*, **44(6)**, 237-241.

Butler, R.J., Redfern, E.J. & Forsythe, I. (1993) Case histories and shorter communications: the Maternal Tolerance Scale and nocturnal enuresis. *Behaviour Research and Therapy*, **31(4)**, 433-436.

Butterfield, P.G. (1990) Thinking upstream: nurturing a conceptual understanding of the societal context of health behaviour. *Advances in Nursing Science*, **12(2)**, 1-8.

Caspi, A. & Elder, G.H. (1988) Emergent family patterns: the intergenerational construction of problem behaviour and relationships. *Relationships within families: mutual influences* (ed. by R.A. Hinde and J. Stevenson-Hinde), p.218-240. Oxford University Press, New York.

Chang, J. & Phillips, M. (1993) New directions in family therapy. *Therapeutic conversations* (ed. by S. Gilligan and R. Price), p.95-111. Norton, New York.

Chenitz, W.C. (1986) The informal interview. *From practice to grounded theory. qualitative research in nursing* (ed. by W.C. Chenitz and J.M. Swanson), p.79-90. Addison-Wesley Publishing, Menlo Park, CA.

Chisholm, C. (1995) Spreading the net wider: the enuresis service Bedford and Shires Health & Care NHS Trust. *Enuresis Update, Enuresis Resource and Information Centre, Bristol*, **July**, 4-6.

Clarke-Stewart, K.A. (1988) Parents' effects on children's development: a decade of progress? *Journal of Applied Developmental Psychology*, **9**, 41-84.

Clements, S. & Cummings, S. (1991) Helplessness and powerlessness: caring for clients in pain. *Holistic Nursing Practice*, **6(1)**, 76-85.

Cockett, M. & Tripp, J. (1994) *The Exeter family study: family breakdown and its impact on children*, University of Exeter Press, Exeter.

Cohen, T.F. (1993) What do fathers provide? Reconsidering the economic and nurturant dimensions of men as parents. *Men, work, and family* (ed. by J.C. Hood), p.1-22. Sage, Newbury Park, CA.

Compas, B.E., Banez, G.A., Malcarne, V. & Worsham, N. (1991) Perceived control and coping with stress: a developmental perspective. *Journal of Social Issues*, **47(4)**, 23-34.

Connell, J.P. & Wellborn, J.G. (1991) Competence, autonomy, and relatedness: a motivational analysis of self-esteem processes. *Self processes and development: The Minnesota symposia on child psychology. Vol. 23* (ed. by M.R. Gunnar and L.A. Sroufe), p.43-77. Lawrence Erlbaum Associates, Hillsdale, NJ.

Corbin, J. (1986) Coding, writing memos, and diagramming. *From practice to grounded theory: qualitative research in nursing* (ed. by W.C. Chenitz and J.M. Swanson), p.102-119. Addison-Wesley Publishing, Menlo Park, CA.

Couchells, S.M., Johnson, S.B., Carter.R., & Walker, D. (1981) Behavioural and environmental characteristics of treated and untreated enuretic children and matched non-enuretic controls. *Journal of Pediatrics*, **99(5)**, 812-816.

Coutts, L.C. & Hardy, L.K. (1985) *Teaching for health: the nurse as health educator*, Churchill Livingstone, Edinburgh.

Coverman, S. & Sheley, J.F. (1986) Changes in men's housework and child-care time. *Journal of Marriage and the Family*, **48**, 413-422.

Covington, M.V. & Omelich, C.L. (1979) Effort: the double-edged sword in school achievement. *Journal of Educational Psychology*, **71**, 169-182.

Covington, M.V. & Omelich, C.L. (1985) Ability and effort valuation among failure-avoiding and failure-accepting students. *Journal of Educational Psychology*, **77**, 446-459.

Cummings, J.S., Pellegrini, D.S., Notarius, C.I. & Cummings, E.M. (1989) Children's responses to angry adult behaviour as a function of marital distress and history of interparent hostility. *Child Development*, **60**, 1035-1043.

Dallos, R. (1995) Constructing family life: family belief systems. *Understanding the family* (ed. by J. Muncie, M. Wetherell, R. Dallos and A. Cochrane), p.174-211. Sage, London.

Dallos, R. & McLaughlin, E. (1994) *Social problems and the family*, Sage (in association with the Open University), London.

Daly, K. (1993) Reshaping fatherhood: finding the models. *Journal of Family Issues*, **14 (4)**, 510-530.

De Jonge, G.A. (1973) Epidemiology of enuresis: a survey of the literature. *Bladder control and enuresis* (ed. by I. Kolvin, R.C. MacKeith and S.R. Meadow), p.39-46. William Heinemann Medical Books, London.

Deatrick, J.A. & Faux, S.A. (1991) Conducting qualitative studies with children and adolescents. *Qualitative nursing research: a contemporary dialogue* (ed. by J.M. Morse), p.203-223. Sage Publications, Newbury Park, CA.

Demo, D.H. & Acock, A.C. (1993) Family diversity and the division of domestic labour: how much have things really changed? *Family Relations*, **42 (3)**, 323-331.

Denzin, N. (1978) *Sociological methods: a source book*, McGraw-Hill, New York.

Denzin, N.K. & Lincoln, Y.S. (1994) *Handbook of qualitative research*, Sage, London.

Deutsch, F.M., Lussier, J.B. & Servis, L.J. (1993) Husbands at home: predictors of paternal participation in child care and housework. *Journal of Personality and Social Psychology*, **65 (6)**, 1154-1166.

Devlin, J.B. (1991) Prevalence and risk factors for childhood nocturnal enuresis. *Irish Medical Journal*, **84(4)**, 118-120.

Devlin, J.B. & O'Cathain, C. (1990) Predicting treatment outcome in enuresis. *Archives of Disease in Childhood*, **65**, 1158-1161.

Dische, S., Yule, W., Corbett, J. & Hand, D. (1983) Childhood nocturnal enuresis: factors associated with outcome of treatment with an enuresis alarm. *Developmental Medicine and Child Neurology*, **25**, 67-80.

Djurhuus, J.C., Norgaard, J.P. & Rittig, S. (1992) Monosymptomatic bedwetting. *Scandinavian Journal of Urology and Nephrology.Supplementum*, **141**, 7-19.

Dobson, P. (1989) Continence. Easing Childhood Shame. *Nursing Times*, **85(33)**, 79-80.

Dodge, W.F., West, E.F., Bridgforth, E.B. & Trains, L.B. (1970) Nocturnal enuresis in 6- to 10-year-old children. *American Journal of Diseases in Children*, **120**, 32-35.

Doherty, W.J. (1986) Quanta, quarks and families: implications of quantum physics for family research. *Family Process*, **25**, 249-264.

Donley, M.G. (1993) Attachment and the emotional unit. *Family Process*, **32 (1)**, 3-20.

Dowd, T.T. (1991) Discovering older women's experience of urinary incontinence. *Research in Nursing and Health*, **14**, 179-186.

Dunn, J. & Brown, J. (1994) Affect expression in the family, children's understanding of emotions, and their interactions with others. *Merrill-Palmer Quarterly*, **40 (1)**, 120-137.

Dunn, L. (1991) Research alert! Qualitative research may be hazardous to your health. *Qualitative Health Research*, **1(3)**, 388-392.

Edwards, S.D. & van der Spuy, H.J.J. (1985) Hypnotherapy as a treatment for enuresis. *Journal of Child Psychology and Psychiatry and Applied Disciplines*, **26**, 161-170.

Eiberg, H., Berendt, I. & Mohr, I. (1995) Assignment of dominant inherited nocturnal enuresis (ENUR1) to chromosome 13q. *Nature Genetics*, **10**, 354-356.

Eisenberg, N. & Fabes, R.A. (1994) Mothers' reactions to children's negative emotions: relations to children's temperament and anger behaviour. *Merrill-Palmer Quarterly*, **40 (1)**, 138-156.

ERIC, (1993) *Issues in treating childhood enuresis highlighted by health visitors and school nurses in a national poll*, Enuresis Resource Information Centre, Bristol.

Erlandson, D.A., Harris, E.L., Skipper, B.L. & Allen, S.D. (1993) *Doing naturalistic inquiry: a guide to methods*, Sage, Newbury Park CA.

Ewles, L. & Simnett, I. (1992) Using and producing health promotion materials. *Promoting health: a practical guide* (ed. by L. Ewles and I. Simnett), p.226-242. Scutari Press, London.

Faux, S.A., Walsh, M. & Deatrick, J.A. (1988) Intensive interviewing with children and adolescents. *Western Journal of Nursing Research*, **10(2)**, 180-194.

Fergusson, D.M., Horwood, L.J. & Shannon, F.T. (1990) Secondary enuresis in a birth cohort of New Zealand children. *Paediatric and Perinatal Epidemiology*, **4(1)**, 53-63.

Fielding, D. (1980) The response of day and night wetting children and children who wet only at night to retention control training and the enuresis alarm. *Behaviour Research and Therapy*, **18**, 305-317.

Fielding, N. (1993) Qualitative interviewing. *Researching social life* (ed. by N. Gilbert), p.135-153. Sage Publications, London.

Fielding, N.G. & Lee, R.M. (1993) *Using computers in qualitative research*, Sage, London.

Findlay, C. & Salter, A. (1992) *Protecting children and young people*, Churchill Livingstone, Edinburgh.

Fontana, A. & Frey, J.H. (1994) Interviewing: the art of science. *Handbook of qualitative research* (ed. by N.K. Denzin and Y.S. Lincoln), p.361-376. Sage Publications, Thousand Oaks, CA.

Ford, M.E. (1992) *Motivating humans: goals, emotions, and personal agency beliefs*, Sage, London.

Fordham, K.E. & Meadow, S.R. (1989) Controlled trial of standard pad and bell alarm against mini alarm for nocturnal enuresis. *Archives of Disease in Childhood*, **64**, 651-656.

Forsythe, W.I. & Butler, R.J. (1989) Fifty years of enuretic alarms. *Archives of Disease in Childhood*, **64(6)**, 879-885.

Forsythe, W.I. & Redmond, A. (1974) Enuresis and spontaneous cure rate: study of 1129 enuretics. *Archives of Disease in Childhood*, **49**, 259-263.

Foxman, B., Valdez, R.B. & Brook, R.H. (1986) Childhood enuresis: prevalence, perceived impact and prescribed treatments. *Pediatrics*, **77**, 482-487.

Foy, S.S. & Mitchell, M.M. (1990) Factors contributing to learned helplessness in the institutionalized aged: a literature review. *Physical and Occupational Therapy in Geriatrics*, **9(2)**, 1-23.

French, N. (1992) The role of hypnotherapy. *Papers from the second national conference of the Enuresis Resource and Information Centre (1991): a comprehensive approach to nocturnal enuresis* (ed. by P. Dobson), p.36. Enuresis Resource and Information Centre, Bristol.

Fuchs, J. (1987) Use of decisional control to combat powerlessness: the patient with end stage renal disease on dialysis. *ANNA Journal*, **14(1)**, 11-13.

Gecas, V. & Schwalbe, M.L. (1986) Parental behaviour and adolescent self-esteem. *Journal of Marriage and the Family*, **48**, 37-46.

Gelles, R.J. (1995) *Contemporary families: a sociological view*, Sage, Thousand Oaks, CA.

Gerson, E.M. (1984) Qualitative research and the computer. *Qualitative Sociology*, **7(1/2)**, 61-74.

Gibson, L.Y. (1989) Bedwetting: a family's recurrent nightmare. *MCN American Journal of Maternal Child Nursing*, **14(4)**, 270-272.

Gilgun, J.F., Daly, K. & Handel, G. (1992) *Qualitative methods in family research*, Sage, Newbury Park, CA.

Glaser, B. (1978) *Theoretical sensitivity*, Sociology Press, Mill Valley CA.

Glaser, B.G. & Strauss, A.L. (1967) *The discovery of grounded theory*, Aldine, Chicago.

Glicklich, L.B. (1951) An historical account of enuresis. *Pediatrics*, **8**, 859-876.

Goldscheider, F.K. & Waite, L.J. (1991) *New families, no families? The transformation of the American home*, University of California Press, Berkeley, CA.

Graham, H. (1986) *Caring for the family*, Health Education Council Research Report No. 1, London.

Graham, H. (1993) *Hardship and health in women's lives*, Harvester Wheatsheaf, London.

Graham, S. (1990) On communicating low ability in the classroom: bad things good teachers sometimes do. *Attribution theory: applications to achievement, mental health, and interpersonal conflict* (ed. by S. Graham and V.S. Folkes), p.17-36. Lawrence Erlbaum, Hillsdale, NJ.

Gray, M. (1994) Personal experience of conducting unstructured interviews. *Nurse Researcher*, **1(3)**, 65-71.

Grych, J.H. & Fincham, F.D. (1990) Marital conflict and children's adjustment: a cognitive-contextual framework. *Psychological Bulletin*, **108**, 267-290.

Gustafson, R. (1993) Conditioning treatment of children's bedwetting: a follow-up and predictive study. *Psychological Reports*, **72 3(1)**, 923-930.

Haas, L. (1993) Nurturing fathers and working mothers: changing gender roles in Sweden. *Men, work, and family* (ed. by J.C. Hood), p.238-261. Sage, Newbury Park, CA.

Haque, M., Ellerstein, N.S., Gundy, J.H., Shelov, S.P., Weiss, J.C., McIntire, M.S., Olness, K.N., Jones, D.J., Heagarty, M.C. & Starfield, B.H. (1981) Parental perceptions of enuresis: a collaborative study. *American Journal of Diseases in Children*, **135**, 809-811.

Harris, K.M. & Morgan, S.P. (1991) Fathers, sons, and daughters: differential paternal involvement in parenting. *Journal of Marriage and the Family*, **53**, 531-544.

Harvey, L. (1990) *Critical social research*, Unwin Hyman, London.

Hellstrom, A.L., Hansson, E., Hansson, S., Hjalmas, K. & Jodal, U. (1990) Micturition habits and incontinence in 7-year-old Swedish school entrants. *European Journal of Pediatrics*, **149 (6)**, 434-437.

Heron, J. (1991) *Helping the client: a creative practical guide*, Sage Publications, London.

Herzog, A.R., Fultz, N.H., Brock, B.M., Brown, M.B. & Diokno, A.C. (1988) Urinary incontinence and psychological distress among older adults. *Psychology and Aging*, **3(2)**, 115-121.

Herzog, A.R., Fultz, N.H., Normolle, D.P., Brock, B.M. & Diokno, A.C. (1989) Methods used to manage urinary incontinence by older adults in the community. *Journal of the American Geriatrics Society*, **37(4)**, 339-347.

Hetherington, E.M. (1989) Coping with family transitions: winners, losers, and survivors. *Child Development*, **60**, 1-14.

Hetherington, E.M. (1992) Coping with marital transitions: a family systems perspective. *Coping with marital transitions: a family systems perspective* (ed. by E.M. Hetherington and W.G. Clingempeel), p.1-14. University of Chicago Press, Chicago, IL.

Hetherington, E.M. & Parke, R.D. (1993) *Child psychology: a contemporary viewpoint*, McGraw-Hill, New York.

Hewlett, S. (1994) Rheumatology: patients' views of changing disability - rheumatoid arthritis. *Nursing Standard*, **8(31)**, 25-29.

Hewstone, M. & Antaki, C. (1994) Attribution theory and social explanations. *Introduction to social psychology* (ed. by M. Hewstone, W. Stroebe, J.P. Codol and G.M. Stephenson), p.111-114. Blackwell, Oxford.

Hewstone, M., Stroebe, W., Codol, J.P. & Stephenson, G.M. (1994) *Introduction to social psychology*, Blackwell, Oxford.

Hinde, R.A. (1989) Reconciling the family systems and the relationships approaches to child development. *Family systems and life-span development* (ed. by K. Kreppner and R.M. Lerner), p.149-163. Erlbaum, Hillsdale, NJ.

Hinde, R.A. & Stephenson-Hinde, J. (1988) *Relationships within families: mutual influences*, Oxford University Press, New York.

Hiroto, D.S. & Seligman, M.E.P. (1975) Generality of learned helplessness in man. *Journal of Personality and Social Psychology*, **31**, 311-327.

Hjälmås, K. (1992) Urinary incontinence in children: suggestions for definitions and terminology. *Scandinavian Journal of Urology and Nephrology.Supplementum*, **141**, 1-6.

Hjälmås, K. & Bengtsson, B. (1993) Efficacy, safety, and dosing of Desmopressin for nocturnal enuresis in Europe. *Clinical Pediatrics*, **July**, 19-24.

Hochschild, A. & Machung, A. (1989) *The second shift: working parents and the revolution at home*, Viking, New York.

Hoffman, L.W. (1989) Effects of maternal employment in the two-parent family. *American Psychologist*, **44 (2)**, 283-292.

Holland, A.M. (1994) Father-child relationships: the issue of discipline. *Australian Journal of Marriage and Family*, **15 (1)**, 15-22.

Hood, J.C. (1993) *Men, work, and family*, Sage, Newbury Park, CA.

Huber, G.L. & Garcia, C.M. (1991) Computer assistance for testing hypotheses about qualitative data: the software package AQUAD 3.0. *Qualitative Sociology*, **14**, 325-348.

Hunskaar, S. & Vinsnes, A. (1991) The quality of life in women with urinary incontinence as measured by the sickness impact profile. *Journal of the American Geriatrics Society*, **39(4)**, 378-382.

Ishii-Kuntz, M. (1993) Japanese fathers: work demands and family roles. *Men, work, and family* (ed. by J.C. Hood), p.45-67. Sage, Newbury Park, CA.

Jarvelin, M.R. (1989) Developmental history and neurological findings in enuretic children. *Developmental Medicine and Child Neurology*, **31(6)**, 728-736.

Jarvelin, M.R., Vikevainen-Tervonen, L., Malanen, I. & Huttunen, N.P. (1988) Enuresis in seven-year-old children. *Acta Paediatrica Scandinavica*, **77**, 148-153.

Jarvelin, M.R., Moilanen, I., Vikevainen-Tervonen, L. & Huttunen, N.P. (1990) Life changes and protective capacities in enuretic and non-enuretic children. *Journal of Child Psychology and Psychiatry and Applied Disciplines*, **31(5)**, 763-774.

Jarvelin, M.R., Moilanen, I., Kangas, P., Moring, K., Vikevainen-Tervonen, L., Huttunen, N.P. & Seppanen, J. (1991) Aetiological and precipitating factors for childhood enuresis. *Acta Paediatrica Scandinavica*, **80(3)**, 361-369.

Jick, T.D. (1983) Mixing qualitative and quantitative methods: triangulation in action. *Qualitative methodology* (ed. by J. Van Maanen), p.135-148. Sage, Beverly Hills, CA.

Johnsen, O. (1992) Different concepts of enuresis nocturna and the practical management within a Danish community. *Papers from the second national conference of the Enuresis Resource and Information Centre (1991): a comprehensive approach to nocturnal enuresis* (ed. by P. Dobson), p.20-25. Enuresis Resource and Information Centre, Bristol.

Jones, S. (1985) Depth interviewing. *Applied qualitative research* (ed. by R. Walker), p.45-55. Gower, Aldershot.

Jorgenson, J. (1989) Where is the "family" in family communication? Exploring families' self definitions. *Journal of Applied Communication Research*, **17**, 27-41.

Kaplan, R.M. (1991) Health-related quality of life in patient decision making. *Journal of Social Issues*, **47(4)**, 69-90.

Kaplan, S.L., Breit, M., Gauthier, B. & Busner, J. (1989) A comparison of three nocturnal enuresis treatment methods. *Journal of the American Academy of Child and Adolescent Psychiatry*, **28(2)**, 282-286.

Karandikar, S. (1992) A comparative study of nocturnal enuresis in Asian and Caucasian four year old children. *Papers from the second national conference of the Enuresis Resource and Information Centre (1991): a comprehensive approach to nocturnal enuresis* (ed. by P. Dobson), p.58-70. Enuresis Resource and Information Centre, Bristol.

Kelley, S.J. (1986) Learned helplessness in the sexually abused child. *Issues in Comprehensive Pediatric Nursing*, **9(3)**, 193-207.

Knafl, K.A. & Webster, D.C. (1988) Managing and analyzing qualitative data: a description of tasks, techniques and materials. *Western Journal of Nursing Research*, **10**, 195-218.

Kohen, D.P. (1991) Applications of relaxation and mental imagery (self hypnosis) for habit problems. *Pediatric Annals*, **20(3)**, 136-144.

Kvale, S. (1995) The social construction of validity. *Qualitative Inquiry*, **1(1)**, 19-40.

Lagro-Janssen, T.L.M., Smits, A.J.A. & Weel, C.V. (1990) Women with urinary incontinence: self-perceived worries and general practitioners' knowledge of problem. *British Journal of General Practice*, **40**, 331-334.

Lamborn, S.D., Mounts, N.S., Steinberg, L. & Dornbusch, S.M. (1991) Patterns of competence and adjustment among adolescents from authoritative, authoritarian, indulgent and neglectful families. *Child Development*, **62**, 1049-1065.

Larsen, K.N., Tarp, M. & Mogensen, H.B. (1992) Application and evaluation of the Danish system. *Papers from the second national conference of the Enuresis Resource and Information Centre (1991): a comprehensive approach to nocturnal enuresis* (ed. by P. Dobson), p.26-31. Enuresis Resource and Information Centre, Bristol.

Larsen, S. & Winther, B. (1980) Work conditions, social status and sex differences, in primary and secondary enuresis. *Scandinavian Journal of Psychology*, **21**, 33-43.

Lazarus, R.S. (1991) *Emotion and adaptation*, Oxford University Press, New York.

Lee, R.M. & Fielding, N.G. (1993) Computing for qualitative research: options, problems and potential. *Using computers in qualitative research* (ed. by N.G. Fielding and R.M. Lee), p.1-13. Sage, London.

Leenders, F.M. (1993) *Social construction of nocturnal enuresis*, Unpublished MSc Thesis, South Bank University, London.

Lefcourt, H.M. (1992) Durability and impact of the locus of control construct. *Psychological Bulletin*, **112(3)**, 411-414.

Leininger, M.M. (1985) Nature, rationale, and importance of qualitative research methods in nursing. *Qualitative research methods in nursing* (ed. by M.M. Leininger), p.1-25. Grune and Stratton, Orlando, FL.

Leyens, J.P. & Codol, J.P. (1994) Social cognition. *Introduction to social psychology* (ed. by M. Hewstone, W. Stroebe, J.P. Codol and G.M. Stephenson), p.89-110. Blackwell, Oxford.

Lincoln, Y.S. & Guba, E.G. (1985) *Naturalistic inquiry*, Sage, Beverly Hills, CA.

Mackaulay, A.J., Stern, R.S. & Stanton, S.L. (1991) Psychological aspects of 211 female patients attending a urodynamic unit. *Journal of Psychosomatic Research*, **35(1)**, 1-10.

Malone-Lee, J. (1992) Some observations of nocturnal enuresis in adolescents and young adults. *Papers from the second national conference of the Enuresis Resource and Information Centre (1991): a comprehensive approach to nocturnal enuresis* (ed. by P. Dobson), p.7-9. Enuresis Resource and Information Centre, Bristol.

Marshall, C. & Rossman, G.B. (1995) *Designing qualitative research*, Sage, Thousand Oaks, CA.

May, K.A. (1991) Interview techniques in qualitative research: concerns and challenges. *Qualitative nursing research: a contemporary dialogue* (ed. by J.M. Morse), p.188-201. Sage Publications, Newbury Park CA.

McDowell, I. & Newell, C. (1987) *Measuring health: a guide to rating scales and questionnaires*, Oxford University Press, Oxford.

Meadow, R. (1977) How to use buzzer alarms to cure bed-wetting. *British Medical Journal*, **ii**, 1073-1075.

Meadow, S.R. (1989) *Desmopressin in nocturnal enuresis*, Horus Medical Publication, London.

Meadow, S.R. (1990) Day wetting. *Pediatric Nephrology*, **4**, 178-184.

Menaghan, E.G. & Parcel, T.L. (1990) Parental employment and family life: research in the 1980s. *Journal of Marriage and the Family*, **52**, 1079-1098.

Mennen, F.E. & Meadow, D. (1994) Depression, anxiety, and self esteem in sexually abused children. *Families in Society*, **75 (2)**, 74-81.

Miles, M.B. & Huberman, A.M. (1994) *Qualitative data analysis: a new source book of methods*, Sage, Newbury Park, CA.

Miller, K., Atkin, B. & Moody, M.L. (1992) Drug therapy for nocturnal enuresis. Current treatment recommendations. *Drugs*, **44(1)**, 47-56.

Minni, B., Capozza, N., Creti, G., DeGennaro, M., Caione, P. & Bischko, J. (1990) Bladder instability and enuresis treated by acupuncture and electro-therapeutics: early urodynamic observations. *Acupuncture and Electro-therapeutics Research*, **15(1)**, 19-25.

Minuchin, P. (1985) Families and individual development: provocations from the field of family therapy. *Child Development*, **56**, 289-302.

Minuchin, P. (1988) Relationships within the family: a systems perspective on development. *Relationships within families: mutual influences* (ed. by R.A. Hinde and J. Stevenson-Hinde), p.7-26. Oxford University Press, New York.

Mitchell, E.S. (1986) Multiple triangulation: a methodology for nursing science. *Advances in Nursing Science*, **8(3)**, 18-26.

Moffatt, M.E., Kato, C. & Pless, I.B. (1987) Improvements in self-concept after treatment of nocturnal enuresis: randomised controlled trial. *Journal of Pedriatrics*, **110(4)**, 647-652.

Moreton, J. (1989) Nocturnal enuresis. *Practice Nurse*, **Nov.**, 260-262.

Morgan, R. (1978) Relapse and therapeutic response in the conditioning treatent of enuresis: a review of recent findings on intermittent reinforcement, overlearning and stimulus intensity. *Behaviour Research and Therapy*, **16**, 273-279.

Morgan, R. (1981) *Childhood incontinence: a guide to problems of wetting and soiling for parents and professionals*, Heinemann Medical Books, London.

Morgan, R. (1988) *Help for the bedwetting child*, Methven, London.

Morgan, R. (1993) *Guidelines on minimum standards of practice in the treatment of enuresis*, Enuresis Resource Information Centre, Bristol.

Morgan, R.T.T. & Young, G.C. (1975) Parental attitude and the conditioning treatment of childhood enuresis. *Behaviour Research and Therapy*, **13**, 197-199.

Morison, M.J. (1995) *Family perspectives on bed wetting in young people*, Unpublished PhD Thesis, Queen Margaret College, Edinburgh.

Morse, J.M. (1991a) The structure and function of gift giving in the patient-nurse relationship. *Western Journal of Nursing Research*, **13(5)**, 597-615.

Morse, J.M. (1991b) Analysing unstructured interactive interviews using the Macintosh computer. *Qualitative Health Research*, **1(1)**, 117-122.

Morse, J.M. (1992) Editorial: The power of induction. *Qualitative Health Research*, **2(1)**, 3-6.

Muncie, J., Wetherell, M., Dallos, R. & Cochrane, A. (eds) (1995) *Understanding the family*, Sage, London.

Murphey, D.A. (1992) Constructing the child: relations between parents' beliefs and child outcomes. *Developmental Review*, **12**, 199-232.

Mussen, P.H., Conger, J.J., Kagan, J. & Huston, A.C. (1990) *Child development and personality*, Harper and Row, New York.

Noller, P. (1994) Relationships with parents in adolencence: process and outcome. *Personal relationships during adolescence: advances in adolescent development Vol.6* (ed. by R. Montemayor, G.R. Adams and T.P. Gullotta), p.37-77. Sage, Thousand Oaks, CA.

Norgaard, J.P. (1991) Pathophysiology of nocturnal enuresis. *Scandinavian Journal of Urology and Nephrology.Supplementum*, **140**, 1-35.